Lippincott Williams & Wilkins'

Pocket Guide for
Medical Assisting

SECOND EDITION

Lippincott Williams & Wilkins'

Pocket Guide for
Medical Assisting

SECOND EDITION

Elizabeth A. Molle, MS, RN
Nurse Educator
Middlesex Hospital
Middletown, Connecticut

Judy Kronenberger, RN, CMA, MEd
Assistant Professor
Sinclair Community College
Dayton, Ohio

Connie West-Stack, AAS (MLT), BS, MEd, CMA
South Piedmont Community College
Monroe, North Carolina

Laura Southard Durham, BS, CMA
Medical Assisting Program Coordinator
Forsyth Technical Community College
Winston-Salem, North Carolina

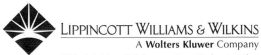

LIPPINCOTT WILLIAMS & WILKINS
A **Wolters Kluwer** Company

Philadelphia • Baltimore • New York • London
Buenos Aires • Hong Kong • Sydney • Tokyo

Acquisitions Editor: John Goucher
Managing Editor: Kevin Dietz
Marketing Manager: Hilary Henderson
Production Editor: Bill Cady
Designer: Risa Clow
Compositor: Graphic World
Printer: R. R. Donnelley & Sons

Printed in the United States of America

First Edition, 1999

ISBN   0-7817-5117-9

To purchase additional copies of this book, call our customer service department
at **(800) 638-3030** or fax orders to **(301) 824-7390.** International customers should
call **(301) 714-2324.**

Visit Lippincott Williams & Wilkins on the Internet: http://www.LWW.com.
Lippincott Williams & Wilkins customer service representatives are available
from 8:30 am to 6:00 pm, EST.

04 05 06 07 08
1 2 3 4 5 6 7 8 9 10

Preface

Lippincott Williams & Wilkins' Pocket Guide for Medical Assisting is designed to help make the transition from class to clinic as smooth and stress-free as possible. The procedures outlined in these pages support theory learned in the classroom as it is transferred to the clinical setting. This pocket-sized guide is not meant to be a stand-alone text but was conceived to be used as a memory aid after you have established proficiency inside a classroom. It is portable, fits easily in a lab coat pocket, and will enhance your externship and postgraduate experiences. Although this book was written as an ancillary to *Lippincott Williams & Wilkins' Textbook for Medical Assistants*, it may be used in conjunction with any comprehensive medical assisting text.

Lippincott Williams & Wilkins' Pocket Guide for Medical Assisting is arranged conveniently in alphabetical order into three sections: Administrative Procedures, Clinical Procedures, and Laboratory Procedures. You will find the procedures are in a logical flow under chapter titles such as "Keeping Track of Finances," "Collecting Payments," "Aseptic Procedures," "Assessment Procedures," and so on. Most procedures include the following elements:

- Title: Alerts you to the name of the procedure
- List of equipment: Outlines the general needs for the particular procedure
- Steps: Lists in logical order the measures needed to complete the procedure successfully
- Purposes for steps: Explains why the steps should be followed
- Warning! Describes special situations that may pose an increased risk to you or your patient
- You Need to Know: Presents what might happen in certain situations or provides adjustments to procedures so you can individualize them for specific patients or circumstances
- Instruct the Patient or Caregiver: Notes how to make at-home care easier for the patient in readily understood terms
- Document on the Patient's Chart: Outlines what should be noted in the patient's chart after performance of the procedure
- Charting Example: Provides a working example of the information required for legal documentation, using several accepted formats
- Procedure Notes: Allows space for you to add points that you encounter in your office setting

Line drawings and photographs are included as needed for clarity and to illustrate points needing visual reinforcement. Boxes and tables are used to remind you of vitally important information. Icons are used to denote procedures that may include a biohazard risk and to remind you to observe Standard Precautions to protect yourself, your patient, and your coworkers. Icons are included for handwashing (soapy hands), gloving (gloves), personal protective equipment (PPE logo), and bio-hazardous containers (biohazard symbol). Normal laboratory test values are located on the inside back cover for easy reference. In Appendix II, you will find a list of common documentation abbreviations.

It is our hope that *Lippincott Williams & Wilkins' Pocket Guide for Medical Assisting* will help make your transition from student to full-fledged professional less stressful. Consider this as "confidence in your pocket."

Elizabeth A. Molle, MS, RN
Judy Kronenberger, RN, CMA, MEd
Connie West-Stack, AAS (MLT), BS, MEd, CMA
Laura Southard Durham, BS, CMA

Contents

Contents

Contents

Contents

LABORATORY PROCEDURES

Contents

Getting Started in Medical Assisting

Congratulations, today you start your externship!

Procedure 1-1

Ensuring a Successful Externship

1. Know your responsibilities:
   - Be dependable.
   - Demonstrate professionalism.
   - Be well groomed and dress in accordance with the office policy.

2. Be prepared. Make sure that you have made arrangements for any personal obligations that you may have (e.g., childcare). Arrange for dependable transportation ahead of time; do not leave this until the night before you begin!

3. Be punctual. Arrive at least 10 minutes early to allow time to get settled before actually starting the day's work. If you are going to be absent for any reason, call the externship site; leave your name, supervisor's name, school's name, and approximate length of time that you will be absent. Depending on school policy, you also may need to call your program instructor.

   Externship site's telephone number: _____
   Preceptor's name: _____

4. Demonstrate a positive attitude and an interest in learning. Whenever possible, anticipate needs and offer to help staff members.

5. Keep records of your time. Depending on policy, your supervisor may need to sign your time sheets. Submit these to the school in a timely manner. Generally, time sheets are mailed weekly, but check your school policy.

6. Complete the site evaluation, and make sure that your professional or student evaluation is completed and submitted to your school. Let the supervisor know that it should be directed to the attention of: _____.

Procedure Notes:

How do you find a permanent position?

Procedure 1-2

Getting a Job

I. Set your goals. On a sheet of paper, describe your ideal job. Include such things as specialty area, duties that you would and would not like to do, type of facility, type of employer and supervisor, desired atmosphere, ideal hours, availability of flextime.

2. Analyze yourself. Be honest. Make a list of your strengths and weaknesses.

3. Search for employment openings. Remember, networking is essential. Start with your externship supervisor or preceptor. Ask for employment leads. Also try placement offices, state and federal employment offices, school placement departments, temporary agencies, and newspapers. Surf the Internet for your local hospital human resources department.

4. Obtain at least three references. Create a document with their names, titles, addresses, and phone numbers.

5. Create a professional resume that is up to date and accurate.

6. Respond to all possible positions with a resume and a cover letter. Watch your spelling!

7. Complete an application. Use only a pen. Print neatly.

8. Prepare for the interview.

9. After the interview, write a thank-you letter and mail it in a timely fashion.

10. If you do not get the job, consider the possible reasons why, then strive to correct any problems.

Procedure Notes:

ADMINISTRATIVE PROCEDURES

2

A Day in the Life of an Administrative Medical Assistant

What must you remember to do when opening the office?

Procedure 2-1

Opening the Office

Did you remember to . . .

1. Unlock all appropriate doors?
2. Disengage the alarm system?
3. Call the answering service to alert them that the office is open and to collect any after-hours messages?
4. Obtain messages from voice mailboxes, e-mail sites, and fax machines?
5. Check the late-night pickup specimen boxes to ensure that items were picked up?
6. Print a computer list of appointments scheduled for the day, or copy the schedule book and supply the appropriate staff with copies?
7. Pull the scheduled patient charts and place them in chronological order?
8. Restock your desk with papers, pens, special forms, and supplies?

2

9. Turn on the lights for the reception area and tidy the reception area as needed?

Procedure Notes:

You Need to Know:

- As the day continues, your responsibilities may include welcoming patients and visitors, registering and orienting new patients, managing telephone calls, and scheduling appointments. Check with your supervisor for a complete list of your responsibilities.

How do you handle routine incoming telephone calls?

Procedure 2-2

Handling Routine Calls

1. Answer all incoming calls with a professional, welcoming voice. If you need to place an incoming call on hold, answer the phone, "Hello, how may I help you?" Then politely ask the caller if you may put him or her on hold. Place the call on hold, but return to it as soon as possible. If an emergency is occurring in the office, return to the caller, ask for his or her name and phone number, and state that you will call back within a certain time frame, for example, 15 minutes.

2. Transcribe all diagnostic laboratory results onto an appropriate form and give them to the proper reviewer (nurse, physician), along with the patient's chart. If the results are stat, give them immediately to the reviewer. To make it easier to document the results, keep copies of laboratory slips at your desk so you can easily fill in the appropriate blanks as the information is relayed to you.

3. Follow the office policy for giving out information regarding patient results. Most offices allow the medical assistant to give out favorable results, but double-check your office policy. Be sure to protect patient confidentiality.

4. If a patient calls the office requesting a prescription refill, take a message regarding the name of the requested medication, the name of the pharmacy, and the patient's name. Pull the patient's chart, and check with either the office nurse or physician before calling the medication in to the pharmacy.

5. Ask sales representatives to leave their names and numbers. If appropriate, you may ask them to call back at a designated time or ask them to send printed information to the office for review.

6. Put through personal calls for physicians as directed by office policy. Most physicians have direct lines with voice mail.

7. Limit your personal calls to break times and personal emergencies.

Procedure Notes:

How do you handle incoming emergency calls?

Procedure 2-3

Telephone Triage

1. Follow your office policy regarding handling medical emergencies. In general, any patient calling the office complaining of chest pain, shortness of breath, loss of consciousness, profuse bleeding, severe vomiting or diarrhea, or temperatures greater than 102°F should be put through to the office nurse or physician.

2. Always obtain the patient's name, address, and phone number so that if you lose the connection, help can be

2

obtained. (Important: The types of emergencies vary greatly among medical specialties. Have your employer write a policy regarding handling such calls.)

3. Provide reassurance to the caller. Remain calm.

4. Keep a telephone log to document all patient triage calls. It should include the date and time of the call, caller's name, patient's name if different, nature of the call, and any information or instructions given to the caller. It is also a good idea to document to whom the call was directed (e.g., Dr. Stricker) and what time he or she returned the call. This allows you to double-check that all patient calls were returned

Procedure Notes:

You Need to Know:

• If you are alone in the office, you should direct the caller to call the Emergency Medical Services number and go to the Emergency Department for evaluation.

How do you call for an ambulance?

Procedure 2-4

Dialing Emergency Medical Services Number
Obtain the following information before dialing: patient's name, age, sex, nature of the medical problem, type of service that is needed, and any special request or instructions from the physician. Make sure that you know the address of the office and any special instructions for the ambulance driver.

1. Dial 9-1-1 or other EMS number.

2. Calmly provide the dispatcher with the above information. Answer the dispatcher questions clearly, concisely, and professionally.

3. Follow the dispatcher's instructions. Do not hang up until directed to do so by the dispatcher.

4. Tell the physician when you have completed the above steps, and give the physician any special information that the dispatcher told you.

Procedure Notes:

You Need to Know:

- After completing the above steps, make sure that the ambulance crew has a clear and direct path into the office. Remove any toys or other obstructions from the path.

- Reassure patients in the waiting room. Maintain patient confidentiality.

- Offer assistance and reassurance to any family members who accompanied the patient to the office.

- Copy any patient forms or documents as directed and place them in an envelope for the ambulance crew.

How do you handle scheduling patient office visits?

Procedure 2-5

Scheduling Routine Patient Appointments

1. Assemble this equipment:
   - Computer and software or files as needed
   - Appointment book
   - Pencil, if manual

2. Obtain the patient's name, and verify whether this is a returning patient or a new patient.

3. Determine the urgency and type of visit needed.

4. Review the open appointments, select possible dates and times, and offer various choices to the patient. Select a date and time.

2

5. Either write the patient's name in the appointment book, or type the patient's name into the computer. Include the reason for the visit or chief complaint and a phone number at which the patient can be reached to confirm the appointment.

6. Answer any patient questions, and restate the date and time of the appointment. If the patient is in the office, complete an appointment card and give it to the patient.

7. If this is a new patient, obtain consent to receive his or her medical records.

Procedure Notes:

WARNING!

You must obtain the patient's consent before requesting that medical records be sent to your office.

You Need to Know:

- When scheduling a new patient, follow all of the above steps, plus provide directions to the office and ask the patient to arrive 10 to 15 minutes early to complete necessary forms. Some offices may mail these papers to the patient to save office time. In this case, include an office orientation brochure.
- Before actually scheduling patients, a matrix must be created. The matrix is created the first time a particular schedule is used, or if changes must be made to the regular matrix.
- A matrix indicates nonavailable office time.
- Be aware that you must note in the patient's chart any missed appointments (Figure 2-1).

Instruct the Patient Regarding:

- The practice's payment policy
- The type of health care provider he or she will be seeing
- The practice's policy on canceling or rescheduling appointments

10/12/04	Patient was scheduled for a routine physi-	
3:30 PM	cal examination today at 9:30 AM. Pt.	**2**
	missed appointment. Pt. was contacted	
	via telephone and stated that she forgot.	
	New appointment set for 10/20/04 at 2 PM.	
	_____ L. Golet, CMA	

Figure 2-1. Charting example for a missed patient appointment.

How do you handle incoming mail?

Procedure 2-6

Opening and Sorting Incoming Mail

1. Assemble this equipment:
   - Letter opener
   - Paperclips
   - Date stamp

2. Open each letter and check for enclosures. Paperclip enclosures to the letter. If the letter states that enclosures were sent, but they are not in the envelope, contact the sender and request them. Indicate on the letter that the enclosures were missing and the name of the person you contacted.

3. Date-stamp each item.

4. Sort the mail into categories and handle appropriately. Paperclip patient test results to the patient's chart, and place the chart on the physician's desk for review. Record insurance payments and checks promptly, and deposit them according to office policy. Account for drug samples, and appropriately log them according to office policy. Dispose of miscellaneous advertisements, unless otherwise directed.

5. Distribute the mail to the appropriate staff members.

Procedure Notes:

Writing a Business Letter

WARNING!

Never allow mail to collect in a mailbox for more than 1 day. If the office is closed, someone should be assigned to pick up the mail, or it should be held at the post office.

You Need to Know:

- If the recipient of urgent mail is on vacation or will be unable to review the mail in a timely manner, bring the urgent letter to the attention of another appropriate staff member.
- If a letter states that correspondence is to be mailed at a later date, place a copy of the letter in your tickler file so you can check that the item arrives as promised.

How do you create and mail a business letter?

Procedure 2-7

Writing a Business Letter

1. Assemble this equipment:
   - Outline notes
   - Pencil or pen
   - Computer and printer
   - Paper

2. Prepare your message by asking yourself these four questions: Who is my reader? What do I want my reader to do? What do I want to say? How will I organize my letter?

3. Access your computer and select the appropriate software program. Open a new document and label it. Select a letter template and an appropriate font.

4. If you do not have access to a computer template program, you will need to insert the elements in Box 2-1, Elements of a Business Letter.

5. Print a draft of the letter. Edit the letter. Look for errors in content, accuracy, grammar, capitalization, punctuation, and spelling. Correct the errors.

6. Insert letterhead stationery into the printer. Print the final copy.

BOX 2-1

Elements of a Business Letter

- Margins—standard margin is 1 inch.
- Today's date, including the month, day, and year. Position the date two to four spaces below the letterhead, or 15 spaces below the top of the page if no letterhead is used. Place the date on one line only, and use no abbreviations.
- Inside address two to four spaces down from the date. (Inside address is the name and address of the person to whom the letter is being sent.) If the letter is going to an individual at his or her place of business, the name of the addressee will be followed by his or her title, the business name, and then the address.
- Subject line three lines below the inside address. It is typed as Re: then the subject of the letter. Keep the subject line to two or three words. (The subject is considered optional. Follow your physician's preference.)
- Salutation two spaces below the previous line. Capitalize the first letter of each word, and follow the phrase with a colon (:). Spell out the word "Doctor." The salutation can be deleted if the letter is informal or if the subject line has been used.
- Body of the letter. Lines are single-spaced, paragraphs are double-spaced.
- Closing, two spaces below the last line of the letter. Capitalize only the first word; follow the closing with a comma (,).
- Leave four spaces for the signature, and type out the name of the sender, along with his or her title.
- Identification line, which consists of initials only. Capitalize the sender's initials, and lower-case the typist's initials.
- Use Enc. (if there is an enclosure) two spaces below the identification line. The number of enclosures is included in parentheses; if only one page is enclosed, just the abbreviation Enc. is used.
- The letter c, indicating a copy, two spaces below the enclosure line, with initials of the recipients. This indicates that a duplicate letter has been sent to someone.

2

2

BOX 2-2

Typing an Envelope

- Type the return address in the upper left-hand corner.
- Type the recipient's address 12 spaces from the top of the envelope.
- Type any special notations; for example, "Personal and confidential" should be typed two spaces below the return address.

7. Select the appropriate template for typing envelopes, and print the envelope.

8. If you do not have access to a computer template program, you will need to insert the elements in Box 2-2 for addressing envelopes.

9. Paperclip the letter and envelope together. Place them in an appropriate place for the sender to see it, read it, and sign it.

10. Copy the final signed letter, and file appropriately.

11. Select the appropriate type of mail service. Affix stamps or labels, and deposit the letter in the postal box.

Procedure Notes:

You Need to Know:

- Use only commonly accepted abbreviations. Never abbreviate business titles when typing the inside address.
- Use spell check with caution! It will highlight misspelled—*not* misused—words.
- If you are instructed to sign a letter for the sender, sign his or her name followed by a slash and your name. Example: Benjamin William, MD/Jason Stricker, CMA.

- If the letter requires more than one page, use letterhead stationery only for the first page. On subsequent pages, type the addressee's name, title, page number, date, and subject on the seventh line from the top. Continue typing the body of the letter three lines down.

WARNING!

All letters created regarding patient information must be copied and added to the patient's permanent medical record.

How would you turn a dictated message into a written format?

Procedure 2-8

Transcribing a Document

1. Assemble this equipment:
   - Transcription machine
   - Headphones
   - Transcription (dictation) tapes
   - Computer
   - Printer

2. Select a transcription tape. Keep in mind that urgent codes must be typed first. If there are no urgent codes, select the tape that has the oldest date.
   Ensures most critical tapes are done first

3. Turn on the transcriber, insert the tape, and rewind it.
   Ensures power availability

4. Put on the headset, and position the foot pedal in a comfortable location.

5. Play a sampling of the tape. Adjust the volume, speed, and tone dials to your comfort.

6. Set appropriate format, and place proper patient identification on the paper.
   Professional appearance for finished document

7. Play a segment of the tape, stop the tape, and type the message. As you gain speed and your skills increase, you will not need to stop the tape.

2

8. If you come across an unfamiliar term, leave a blank space in the document and continue transcribing. After you have finished the document, check with a colleague for clarification.

9. When you have finished, place the initials of the provider, followed by a slash and your initials on the bottom of the page. Then type the date.

10. Spell-check the document.

11. Print and proofread the document.

12. Leave the document and the tape in a designated area for review. After the provider has reviewed and approved the document, make a copy of it and place it in the patient's chart.

13. Send the report to the recipient.

14. Erase the tape and return to the dictation area.

15. Turn off the power to the equipment, and return it to its proper place.

Procedure Notes:

WARNING!

Never erase a tape until the person who dictated it has read and approved the printed copy.

How can you make the most of your computer?

Procedure 2-9

Electronic Mail

1. Assemble this equipment:
   - Computer with appropriate software program
   - Modem

2. Access your e-mail account.

3. To read a message, click on the message and read it. Respond promptly. If the message is not something you can address, forward it to the appropriate person.

4. To send e-mail, type in the address of one or more recipients, type the message, edit it, spell-check the message, and then click on the send button. Be sure the address is correctly typed. (Note: It is possible to send patients' charts, laboratory results, or other diagnostic information via e-mail, but you must be careful to protect patient confidentiality.)

5. Delete messages that do not need to be saved. Place other messages into appropriate folders.

6. If you are going to be out of the office for more than 1 day, turn on the automatic out-of-office assistant. Your message should include a date and time for your return and a name and e-mail address of someone to whom messages should be rerouted.

Procedure Notes:

WARNING!

- Do not give your password to anyone. Create a password that is unique. Do not use your initials. A combination of letters and numbers is best.
- Do not put your password on a piece of paper and tape it to the computer.
- Do not access anyone else's e-mail messages unless specifically told to do so.
- Use extreme caution when e-mailing confidential patient information. Computer hackers who can access physician and hospital addresses can read protected information.

2

BOX 2-3

Search Engines

Google.com   Excite.com

Yahoo.com   Dogpile.com

Lycos.com

You Need to Know:

- Use the office e-mail only for work-related projects.
- Do not participate in chain letters.
- Do not open any suspicious messages.
- Use your e-mail software's encryption device

How do I use the Internet for work-related information?

Procedure 2-10

Surfing the Internet

1. Assemble this equipment:
   - Computer with appropriate software program
   - Modem
2. Access the Internet.
3. Locate a search engine. See Box 2-3 for some common search engine sites.
4. Select one or two key terms/words and type them at the appropriate space on the web page. Click enter, or click the search button.
5. View the results. If no sites were found, check the spelling or choose another word or phrase. If the search produced a long list, perform an advanced search and refine your key words.
6. Select an appropriate site, and open its home page.
7. Either download the information or bookmark the page for later reference.
8. Exit out of the Internet when the task is completed.

Procedure Notes:

WARNING!

Use only professional medical sites.

You Need to Know:

- Do not use the Internet at work for your own personal use.
- Educate patients about the dangers and benefits of using the Internet for medical information.
- Many excellent sites on the Internet provide great patient education information. Some sites are also in Spanish. Consider updating your patient education pamphlets with Web site addresses.
- List common Web site addresses under "personal modifications" for quick and easy access.

How do you teach patients all they need to know?

Procedure 2-11

Patient Education

1. Determine exactly what the patient needs to know.

2. Ensure that appropriate information and supplies are present, such as videos, pamphlets, and brochures.

3. Identify any factors that may hinder learning, and plan appropriately.

4. Provide the information in a clear, concise, and chronological order.

5. Evaluate the patient's and caregiver's comprehension level.

6. Reinforce the material as needed. Remind the patient to call the office with any questions or concerns.

7. Document all teaching in the patient's medical record.

Procedure Notes:

2

Document on the Patient's Chart:

- Date and time of the teaching
- Names of caregivers who were present
- What was taught
- How it was taught (e.g., verbal instructions, written instructions, demonstration)
- Any materials given to patient
- Patient's level of comprehension
- Follow-up instructions given
- Signature

WARNING!

Teach within your scope of knowledge and practice. Do not guess or provide information that you are not trained in. Refer the patient to the physician or other provider for additional clarification.

You Need to Know:

- Provide education to all available caregivers.
- Stress the importance of routine and preventive medicine
- Use the Internet to get up-to-date patient education materials.
- Call the patient in 2 to 3 days to verify progress and to assist with any problems.

How do you create a file to hold patient information?

Procedure 2-12

Preparing a Medical Record File

1. Assemble this equipment
   - File folder
   - Title, year, and alphabetic or numeric labels
   - Any other labels that your office uses (e.g., insurance information, drug allergies, advance directives)
2. Decide the name of the file (patient's name, company name, or the type of information to be stored within the record). Follow the indexing rules in your textbook.

3. Type a label with the selected title in unit order (e.g., type: Sefferin, Faith, M., not M. Faith Sefferin).

4. Place the label along the tabbed edge of the folder so that the title extends out beyond the folder itself. (Tabs can be placed the length of the folder or tabbed in various positions.)

5. Place a year label along the top edge of the tab, before the label with the title. This is changed each year to indicate that a chart is current. Note: Do not automatically update year stickers until the patient actually comes in to the office for a visit.

6. Place the appropriate alphabetic or numeric labels below the title.

7. Apply any additional labels that your office may decide to use.

Procedure Notes:

WARNING!

Never release any patient information or documentation without the patient's consent and signed release of medical record authorization form

How do you document in a medical record?

Procedure 2-13

Documenting in a Medical Record

1. Assemble this equipment:
   • Patient's chart
   • Black pen
   Note: Some offices have computerized charting systems. In this case, you would need the computer, keyboard, and monitor.

2. Make sure you have the correct chart. Use caution with patients with similar last names.

2

3. Always document in ink; black is preferred.
   Ensures permanence and photocopies are more legible

4. Select the appropriate documentation format, for example, Narrative (Figure 2-2), SOAP (Figure 2-3), PIE (Figure 2-4).

| 05/31/04 8:30 AM | Pt. arrived for BP screening. BP—Left arm 170/80, right arm 165/70. Pt. denies any complaints. States he is taking his BP meds as ordered. Dr. Williams in to see patient.
_____ Sarah Richards, CMA |

Figure 2-2. Narrative charting example.

| 07/12/04 1300 | S: "My leg hurts. I fell yesterday at the beach."
O: Right ankle swollen, tender to touch. Good pedal pulse. Good capillary refill in all toes. No discoloration noted.
A: Injured right ankle
P: Elevate R ankle. Dr. Meza notified and she will be in to see pt.
_____ Brian Sargent, CMA |

Figure 2-3. SOAP charting example.

| 02/02/04 4:00 PM | P: Pt. arrived in office for suture removal.
I: 5 sutures removed from left arm as ordered by Dr. Shea. No s/s of infection. Wound healing nicely. Band-Aid applied to left arm.
E: Pt. denies any questions. Pt. was d/c and told to call office for any additional concerns.
_____ Tim Jones, CMA |

Figure 2-4. PIE charting example.

5. Enter the date and time that the interaction occurred. Military time is considered standard.

2

6. Document all subjective and objective findings, all procedures that you performed, to whom you reported any findings, any patient education, any missed appointments, and any telephone conversations. Use patient quotes whenever possible.

7. Sign your name and title.

Procedure Notes:

You Need to Know:

- Limit the use of abbreviations; they can cause confusion (e.g., BS can mean breath sounds, bowel sounds, or blood sugar).
- Document what honestly happened. If a wrong medication was given, document the facts: "X medication given, Dr. Smith notified."

WARNING!

- *Never document for someone else.*
- *Never document false information.*
- *Never diagnose a condition. For example, do not write "Patient has pharyngitis." Instead write "Patient c/o a sore throat."*
- *Never erase, delete, white out, or scribble over information. Doing so may be construed as tampering with a legal document*

What must you remember to do when closing the office?

Procedure 2-14

Closing the Office

Did you remember to . . .

1. Turn off all electronic equipment?

2. Organize and tidy the reception area?

2

3. Place any specimens for pickup in the night specimen container?

4. Notify the answering service that you are leaving? (Some offices have the answering service automatically turn on, but it is always a good idea to check with the service.)

5. Lock all the doors and close any windows?

6. Arrange for mail to be taken out to the drop box or post office? Arrange for bank deposits to be made?

7. Adjust the air conditioners or set the heat at a reasonable level?

8. Engage the alarm system?

Procedure Notes:

You Need to Know:

• Be aware that your office may have certain policies regarding closing, especially with regard to handling and depositing of cash and payments. Check with your supervisor for a complete list of your responsibilities.

3

Keeping Track of Finances

How would you post a charge on a day sheet?

Procedure 3-1

Posting a Charge

1. Assemble this equipment:
   - Day sheet
   - Pegboard
   - Ledger card
   - Pen or pencil
   - Superbill/encounter form

   Note: Financial records may be kept on a computer. Follow the prompts as instructed.

2. Place a day sheet on the pegboard and enter the date. Align the patient's ledger card (Figure 3-1) on top of the sheet. If the patient was seen in the office, a superbill will be used. Position the superbill appropriately on top of the ledger card. Check to make sure that the ledger line for the current day's charges and the appropriate line on the day sheet exactly correspond.
   Ensures legibility and correct placement

3. Record the patient's name and previous balance in the appropriate columns. If the patient does not have a previous balance, enter 0. If a superbill is used, place the number of the superbill in the appropriate receipt column.
   Enables current balance to be tallied

3

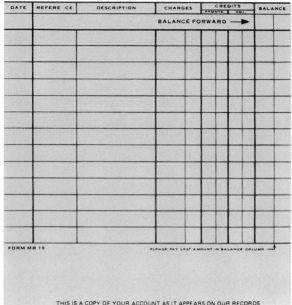

Figure 3-1. Sample ledger card.

4. Record the posting date in the date column. If the date
of the posting is different from the procedure date, indicate the procedure date in the description column.
*Ensures that appropriate information is present for insurance reim-
bursement*

5. Enter the correct procedure code in the description
column.
Provides explanation for charge

6. Enter the total charges for the procedure in the fee
column.
Summarizes total cost for procedure

7. Add the previous balance to the new fee, and record the
current balance in the balance column.
Summarizes most current balance

8. Return the patient's ledger card to the ledger file.
Aids office organization

Procedure Notes:

You Need to Know:

• If a computer system is used, enter the data according to the prompts. Save all data, print a final copy of the transaction, and file it appropriately.

How would you post a credit on a day sheet?

Procedure 3-2

Posting a Credit

I. Assemble this equipment:
   • Day sheet
   • Pegboard
   • Ledger card
   • Pen or pencil
   Note: Financial records may be kept on a computer. Follow the prompts as instructed.

2. Place a fresh day sheet on the pegboard and enter the date. Align the patient's ledger card on top of the sheet. If the patient was seen in the office, a superbill should be used. Position the superbill appropriately on top of the ledger card. Check to make sure that the ledger line for the day's charges and the appropriate line on the day sheet exactly correspond.
   Ensures legibility and correct placement

3. Record the patient's name and previous balance in the appropriate columns.
   Enables current balance to be tallied

4. Enter the amount of the payment in the appropriate column. Subtract the payment from the previous balance. If the result is a negative number, place a minus ($-$) sign in front on the number.
   Confirms that overpayment has been made

3

5. Enter the negative number in the new balance column in brackets, for example, [4.00].

Eliminates confusion regarding a positive or negative balance

6. Enter the bank identification number and the amount of the payment in the appropriate area of the deposit slip. Place the deposit slip and payment in the appropriate place.

Ensures that the payment will be deposited correctly in the bank

Procedure Notes:

WARNING!

It is illegal and unethical to keep overpayments from insurance companies. It also is illegal to delay returning an insurance overpayment. Your office may be fined if overpayments are not returned promptly and accurately.

You Need to Know:

- You can handle overpayments by patients in two ways:
  1. Leave the credit on the patient's account and subtract it from the charges on the patient's next visit.
  2. Mail the patient a refund in the amount of the overpayment.
- The way in which an overpayment is handled depends on the office policy and the amount of overpayment. Generally, overpayments of less than $5.00 are left on account as a credit, whereas overpayments of more than $5.00 are refunded.

How would you post an adjustment on a day sheet?

Procedure 3-3

Posting an Adjustment (Credit or Debit)

1. Assemble this equipment:
- Day sheet
- Pegboard

- Ledger card
- Pen or pencil

Note: Financial records may be kept on a computer. Follow the prompts as instructed.

2. Place a fresh day sheet on the pegboard and enter the date. Align the patient's ledger card on top of the sheet. If the patient was seen in the office, a superbill will be used. Position the superbill appropriately on top of the ledger card. Check to make sure that the ledger line for today's charges and the appropriate line on the day sheet exactly correspond.
Ensures legibility and correct placement

3. Record the patient's name and previous balance in the appropriate columns.
Enables current balance to be tallied

4. Record the type of adjustment in the adjustment column on the ledger card. Examples of credit adjustments may be a professional service charge or an insurance adjustment. If you are making a debit adjustment, you must post it with brackets around the amount, for example, [15.00].
Eliminates confusion regarding a positive or negative balance

5. If you are posting a credit adjustment, subtract the amount of the payment from the previous balance. If you are posting a debit adjustment, add the payment to the previous balance.
Enables current balance to be tallied

Procedure Notes:

How would you post a payment on a day sheet?

Procedure 3-4

Posting a Payment

1. Assemble this equipment:
- Day sheet
- Pegboard

3

• Ledger card
• Pen or pencil

Note: Financial records may be kept on a computer. Follow the prompts as instructed.

2. Place a fresh day sheet on the pegboard and enter the date. Align the patient's ledger card on top of the sheet. If the patient was seen in the office, a superbill will be used. Position the superbill appropriately on top of the ledger card. Check to make sure that the ledger line for today's charges and the appropriate line on the day sheet exactly correspond.

Ensures legibility and correct placement

3. Record the patient's name and previous balance in the appropriate columns. If the patient does not have a previous balance, enter 0. If a superbill is used, place the number of the superbill in the appropriate receipt column.

Enables current balance to be tallied

4. Record the posting date in the date column.

Shows date payment was made

5. Enter the type of payment being made in the appropriate column or in the description column. (Examples: personal check, pers ck; money order, mo; insurance check, ins ck; charge card, chg.) Enter the amount of the payment in the payment column.

Documents payment

6. Subtract the payment amount from the previous balance, and record the new balance in the balance column.

Summarizes patient's current balance

Procedure Notes:

WARNING!

You must immediately place any cash received in a designated secure area. Never leave cash unattended.

4

Collecting Payments

What do you do when a patient's bill is unpaid?

Procedure 4-1

Collecting a Debt

1. Assemble this equipment:
   - Accounting ledger
   - Billing materials
   - Computer or word processor

2. Select a method for debt collection. The three most common methods are sending an overdue notice to the patient, calling the patient, and reminding the patient while he or she is in the office. Be aware that the method used is based on the amount due, tardiness of the debt, and office policy.
   Ensures appropriate collection method is used

3. If you write an overdue notice, be direct but nonthreatening. Offer financial plans for repayment. If you telephone the patient, speak only to the patient or to the designated payer. Be nonthreatening, and offer financial plans for repayment. Do not contact the patient at his or her place of employment. If you remind the patient in the office, be sure the discussion is held privately.
   Shows professionalism, prevents legal complications, protects patient confidentiality

4. Document the method used and any payment plans that have been agreed on.
   Provides record of discussion

Collecting a Debt

Procedure Notes:

4

WARNING!

By law, patients must be alerted to any changes in the facility's billing cycle 3 months before the change takes effect.

You Need to Know:

- If you are collecting a debt from an estate:
  - Never contact the family immediately after the death. Most offices have a policy that states that family members will not be contacted until 2 to 3 weeks after the funeral date.
  - Contact the next of kin and determine who is the executor of the patient's estate. (This may be a friend, spouse, attorney, or some other person.) Contact the executor by letter. Be sure the letter is compassionate, but be direct.
  - Make sure your claim against a patient's estate is made promptly. In case the estate does not have enough funds to meet all of its debts, the local probate court will decide the priority list for debt collection.
  - Be sure to use reasonable restraint when contacting a patient about a bill. Box 4-1 lists some important "don'ts" concerning debt collection.
  - Be aware that collection agencies may also be used. It is important to assess such agencies for integrity and philosophy regarding collections. Most office policies indicate that the physician be alerted about a particular case before it is turned over to a collection agency.

BOX 4-1

Seven Don'ts for Debt Collection

1. Don't contact the patient at his or her place of employment.
2. Don't contact a third party about payment of a debt without court authorization.
3. Don't contact the patient before 8:00 AM or after 9:00 PM.
4. Don't contact the patient at all if the patient has filed for bankruptcy.
5. Don't harass or intimidate the patient, that is, use abusive language, provide false or misleading information, or pose as someone other than a debt collector.
6. Don't threaten to take actions without taking the action.
7. Don't drop the ball. Follow up on unfulfilled promises to pay.

4

How do you code a service so that the practice is reimbursed correctly?

Procedure 4-2

Diagnostic and Procedural Coding

1. Assemble this equipment:
   - CPT coding book
   - ICD-9 coding book
   - Medical terminology book or medical dictionary
   - Form used for service documentation (e.g., superbill, encounter form)

2. Review the superbill form. Check the diagnosis, surgery, or service that was performed. If you are unsure of what the term means, check a medical terminology book for clarification.
   Decreases coding errors caused by lack of understanding

3. Select the appropriate coding book, and then find the appropriate code within the book. Always check for indentations next to the condition for a more accurate

code. ICD-9 is used for disease classifications; CPT is used for procedural and service coding.

Ensures proper code assignment

4. Look at the Health Care Financing Administration's common procedure coding system (HCPCS) for any additional services (e.g., ambulance services, wheelchairs) that are not listed in other texts.

Allows reimbursement of nonphysician services

Procedure Notes:

WARNING!

· Never code directly from the alphabetic index in the ICD-9 book.
· Never submit a claim unless you are sure it is correct. It is always better to ask for help or double-check a code before submitting it.
· It is illegal to bill for services not rendered or to upcode services to receive additional funds. Fraud is a felony!

You Need to Know:

• The ICD-9 book includes three volumes, two of which are used in the outpatient medical facility. Volume 1 contains the classifications of diseases and injuries by code numbers. A code has three digits. Whenever possible, use a subcategory code, which adds an extra digit. A fifth digit may be added to further specify a disorder. In addition, Volume 1 has five appendices. Appendix A is for morphology of neoplasms. It is used in conjunction with Chapter 2 and details neoplasms. Appendix B is used to classify mental disorders. Appendix C is used for the classification of drugs by the American Hospital Formulary Service. Appendix D is used for classifying industrial accidents. These codes are used as supplements for explaining an injury. Appendix E is a list of all three-digit categories that appear in the ICD. Volume 2 is the alphabetical index of diseases. Volume 3 is a tabular list and alphabetic index of procedures based on anatomy, not surgical specialty.

Example of a Health Plan With a PPO		
Benefit	In-network	Out-of-network
Deductible	$100	$300
Coinsurance	90%	70%
Routine care	$200 per calendar year	-0-
Mental health	80%	50%
Office visit	$10 co-pay; no deductible	70%

4

Figure 4-1. CMS 1500 form.

- If you are using the CPT book, remember that the most commonly used section is Evaluation and Management. However, to use this section, you must have two of the three "key components" present. The three key components are history, examination, and medical decision-making.

How do I fill out a medical claim form?

Procedure 4-3

Completing the CMS (Formerly HCFA 1500 Claim Form)

1. Assemble this equipment:
   - CMS claim form (Figure 4-1)

     Note: This form may be submitted electronically, by means of computer and modem, to the clearinghouse, allowing for quicker financial reimbursement. However, it is important to note that electronically submitted claims that do not precisely meet criteria will be rejected by the clearinghouse and must be resubmitted by mail. Claims with multiple attachments must be submitted by mail even if the form is on the computer.

2. Complete each box as defined in Box 4-2. Do not leave empty boxes; place n/a in nonapplicable boxes.

Procedure Notes:

BOX 4-2

Important Information Required on a Medical Claim

Because the CMS 1500 is the claim form most frequently used, it is provided here as the example for completing a claim form. Other claim forms may be in different formats, but will require essentially the same information. A computer is useful and time-saving. Software allows a user to move from field to field, establish default settings, and automatically place information in the appropriate field based on information entered on the patient's first visit. Electronic claims are transmitted across the phone lines or digitally.

Box No.	Information to Be Entered	Comments
1	Where the claim is being submitted	Confirm the patient's coverage and accuracy of your file information. A change in the patient's coverage will change how the claim is filed.
1a	The insured's ID number	Important: It is the ID number of the "Insured" (or "employee"), not the patient, that is required here. This is a frequent filing error and will result in the rejection of the claim. The insured's ID number is often the insured's Social Security number (SSN); check the ID card, the correct ID number required by the company may differ from the SSN.
2	Patient's name	The correct order is important (last, first, middle initial).

Box No.	Information to Be Entered	Comments
3	Patient's birthday	
4	Insured's name	Again, be sure that it is the name of the "insured" (or "employee") that is entered here, not the name of the patient.
5	Address of the patient	
6	Patient relationship to the insured	
7	Address of the insured	Check and update regularly.
8	Patient status	This will need to be checked and updated frequently.
9	Other insured's name	If the patient is covered under more than one plan, the second plan should be entered here. For example, if Jane's claim is being submitted to the insurance company for her employer but she is also covered under her husband Joe's plan, Joe's name would be listed here.
9a	Other insured's policy or group number	Joe's policy number would be entered here.
9b	Other insured's date of birth	Joe's date of birth and sex
9c	Employer's name or school name	The name of Joe's employer

continued

4

Box No.	Information to Be Entered	Comments
9d	Insurance plan name or program name	The name of Joe's insurance company
10	Patient's condition	
10a	Patient's condition related to employment?	If yes, the claim should be submitted to the Workers' Compensation carrier.
10b	Related to an auto accident?	If yes, the claim will not be processed unless a police report is attached.
10c	Other accident?	If yes, details of that accident must be attached for the claim to be processed.
11	Insured's policy group or Federal Employees' Compensation Act (FECA) number	Very important, some payers will automatically return the claim if the group number is not indicated here. The group number is on the patient's ID card.
11a	Insured's date of birth	Again note, this is the insured, not the patient.
11b	Employer's name	The insured's employer or school name
11c	Insurance plan name or program name	
11d	Is there another health plan?	If the patient is covered under more than one plan, check yes. If yes, the coverage will be coordinated between the plans covering the patient.
12	Patient's or authorized person's signature	This signature authorizes the release of information necessary to process the claim. If a release form has been signed and is in the patient file, then "Signature on File" may be entered here.

Box No.	Information to Be Entered	Comments
13	Insured's signature	The signature of the insured
14	Date of current illness or accident	This is not the date of service, but the date the illness began or the accident occurred. If a diagnosis code in the 800-940 range is used, you must list a date of accident.
15	If patient has had same or similar illness	Has the patient had this illness in the past? If so, enter the date the patient first had this illness.
16	Is patient unable to work?	This information is required for the patient to receive disability payments.
17	Name of referring physician	If this patient was referred by another physician, enter that physician's name here.
17a	ID number of referring physician	Enter the Employer ID Number (EIN) of the physician who referred the patient.
18	Hospitalization dates	If the patient has been hospitalized due to this illness or the reason for this visit, enter the dates of the hospitalization here.
20	Outside lab	If lab charges were incurred related to this visit and were provided by an outside lab, check yes and enter the amount of charges. If not, simply check no.
21-24	Codes	The accuracy of the information entered in these sections determines the accuracy of the reimbursement received by the physician. A thorough understanding of coding is essential in completing this section.

4

continued

Box No.	Information to Be Entered	Comments
25	Federal tax ID number	Enter the EIN of the physician.
26	Patient's account number	If you have an account number assigned to the patient, enter that number here.
27	Accept assignment?	If you will accept the fees predetermined by an insurance company, check yes. If not, check no.
28	Total charge	Enter the total amount of charges for this visit or service.
29	Amount paid	Enter here any amount paid by the patient.
30	Balance due	Subtract any amount paid from the total charge and enter that amount here.
31	Signature of physician	
32	Name and address of facility where services were rendered	If the service was rendered outside of the physician's office, enter that address here.
33	Physician's billing name, address, zip code, and phone	This is the information that will be used to mail reimbursement. Be sure it is current. Note that the physician's billing name is required; this may be a practice or corporate name. If so, be sure to enter that billing name here.

5

Managing Employee-Related Issues

What should you remember to do when completing an incident report?

Procedure 5-1

Completing an Incident Report

1. State only the facts. Do not draw conclusions or summarize the event. If you did not see the event, document only the parts that you saw. Use quotation marks when documenting what someone says. For example, write, "Patient states that he tripped in the parking lot" and not "Patient tripped in the parking lot."

2. Write legibly.

3. Do not leave any blank lines or boxes. Insert N/A as needed.

4. Complete the form in a timely fashion; within 24 hours is considered acceptable.

5. Never photocopy the report for your own records.

6. Never place the form inside a medical record file. Document the incident in the chart.

7. Use the correct type of form. Some offices will have separate forms for employee, patient, or visitors.

8. After completing the form, sign it and date it. Submit it to the physician or other designated person. After they have reviewed and signed the form, it should be filed in an appropriate file and used for tracking reasons.

Issuing Payroll Checks

Procedure Notes:

5

You Need to Know:

- Complete an incident report even if no injury occurred. You are documenting an unusual or untoward event (patient fall, needle stick).
- Incident reports should not be considered a punitive report.
- They do not imply wrongdoing. It is a statement of events.

How do you issue a payroll check?

Procedure 5-2

Issuing Payroll Checks

1. Obtain all employee time sheets.
2. Review time sheets for accuracy. Clarify any discrepancies.
3. Calculate employee's earnings. See Box 5-1.
4. Issue checks per office policy.

Procedure Notes:

BOX 5-1

Calculating Employee Earnings

- To calculate the amount of an employee's payroll check, begin by calculating the employee's annual gross wage using the following formula:

  Hourly wage × number of hours worked per week
  × 52 (number of weeks in 1 year)
  = gross annual wage

5

- Assume an employee earns $7.00 per hour and works 40 hours per week:

  $7.00 × 40 × 52 = $14,560 gross annual wage

- If the pay period for your facility is biweekly or monthly, you then divide this sum by 26 or 12, respectively, to calculate this pay period's gross wages.

- What if the employee missed a day during the pay period and you must deduct this? Always start with the normal gross wage (actual earned amount), then deduct a day's pay. To do this, go back to the year's gross amount, divide by 52 (weeks in 1 year), and then divide by 5 (work days in 1 week) to get the amount of 1 day's pay. Deduct this amount from the gross wage to get the adjusted gross wage from which you withhold taxes. Using the example above, the calculation would be as follows:

  ($14,560 ÷ 52) ÷ 5 = day's pay
  $280 ÷ 5 = $56
  $280 − $56 = $224 (adjusted gross wage)

- If you always use the gross annual wage when figuring deductions or increases to gross wages, you will get the exact amount.

continued

5

Calculating Employee Earnings—*cont'd*

- Increases to gross wages may be the overtime worked. Overtime is defined as hours worked over the normal for the pay period. Overtime is calculated as $1\frac{1}{2}$ times the normal hourly wage. If the employee earns $7.00 per hour, overtime pay is calculated by dividing $7.00 in half ($3.50) and adding that amount to the hourly wage; the hourly pay rate for overtime in this case is $10.50.

- Once you have calculated the employee's gross wages, refer to the appropriate tax tables for the deductions for taxes (e.g., federal, FICA/Medicare, state taxes). Subtract the taxes from the gross or adjusted gross wages to obtain net pay. This is the amount for which you write the payroll check.

You Need to Know:

- Paychecks must be kept in a secure location.
- Payroll information involves very confidential information. You have access to each employee's Social Security number. These numbers must be held with the utmost security.
- Never discuss an individual's hourly rate with other staff members.
- If possible, have a separate password for accessing the payroll software program. Always completely exit the computer program when leaving your desk, even if you plan on returning momentarily.
- Be sure that you are using the most recent deduction charts from your state and federal government. Be alert for new regulations regarding payroll deductions.
- Most paycheck stubs have a tally of an employee's vacation, holiday, and sick days. Be sure that these tallies are accurate.

WARNING!

- It is illegal to change a person's deductions without their knowledge and a new signed W-2 form.
- It is illegal to not withhold any deductions.
- Never pay someone or yourself a higher hourly rate than what is signed and agreed to per the employment contract.

What must you remember to do if you are a new medical office manager?

Procedure 5-3

Handling Your Job as the Medical Office Manager

Did you remember to . . .

1. Create a file for each employee, including employment papers, payroll deduction forms, performance appraisals, and letters of recommendation?

2. Create a current and accurate job description for each type of employee?

3. Schedule a regular staff meeting? Create and post agendas? Compose minutes?

4. Develop and maintain a quality improvement program?

5. Conduct or schedule staff in-services? Certify or recertify staff in CPR?

6. Create a standard application form for new employees?

7. Review and update employee orientation and competency forms?

8. Review and update policy and procedure manuals for infection control, employee-related issues, clinical tasks, and administrative duties?

9. Obtain current coding book textbooks and reference manuals?

10. Document all disciplinary actions taken with employees, and document any discussion with a physician regarding the incident?

11. Ensure that all promotional materials are accurate and up to date?

12. Ensure that all educational materials are accurate and up to date?

13. Establish and review the budget regularly, and promptly address any concerns with an appropriate person?

14. Maintain your professional education and affiliations?

15. Keep track of all legal regulations from such entities as your state's medical board, your state's department of public health, OSHA, ADA, CLIA, and CMS?

16. Assign a privacy officer per regulations of the HIPAA? Ensure that the office is in compliance with HIPAA regulations?

5

Procedure Notes:

You Need to Know:

- Federal, state, and local regulations are changed frequently. You are responsible for keeping abreast of new changes, alerting your supervisor or other key personnel to these changes, and implementing them as needed.

CLINICAL PROCEDURES

6

Opening and Closing the Clinical Area

What routine should you follow to open the clinical area of the office?

Procedure 6-1

Opening the Clinical Area

1. Check each room for sufficient patient gowns, drapes, table paper, paper towels, and other supplies.

2. Replace sharps containers that are filled to the caution line. Store used containers in the secure, designated area.

3. Restock all medical and surgical supplies.

4. Ensure that backup supplies are available in each room.

5. Check expiration dates of supplies in each room, and replace as needed.

6. Properly dispose of expired solutions and materials.

7. Check the emergency cart or tray for all needed supplies and equipment. Check the defibrillator, if applicable.

8. Check that each room has a functioning diagnostic set (otoscope and ophthalmoscope). Check for additional batteries and bulbs as needed. Check electronic and tympanic thermometers and all other electronic equipment for function.

6

9. If tables have heating units for specula, turn these on now.

10. If items are to be sterilized from the previous day's procedures, follow the procedure for autoclaving equipment and supplies.

11. Prepare new solutions for disinfection purposes. Clean, sterilize, and replace all containers for wet storage of instruments.

12. Arrange the charts for the day in chronological order if this is not done by the administrative staff.

13. Post your day's clinical schedule in a location that is away from the patient area but available for you to check and update frequently.

14. Check the presenting conditions of your scheduled patients for special equipment and supplies that you will need.

15. Begin to call your patients back to the clinical area.

Note: To save time in the morning, you may prefer to complete some of these tasks before leaving the office each evening.

Procedure Notes:

What steps should be followed to secure the clinical area at the close of the day?

Procedure 6-2

Closing the Clinical Area

1. Check each room for needed supplies and equipment, such as gowns, drapes, table paper, paper towels, and so forth.

2. Plug in the rechargeable units, such as diagnostic sets, electronic thermometers, and so on, for overnight charge.

3. Turn off the electricity to examining tables and electronic equipment.

4. Glove and sanitize instruments used during the day. Wrap them to be autoclaved the next morning.

5. Glove and clean surfaces of counters and examining tables with an environmental disinfectant.

6. With gloves and appropriate PPE, gather biohazard bags and filled sharps containers and place them in the secure designated area for pickup by the biohazard waste service.

7. Bag and discard regular, uncontaminated waste.

8. Double-check the security of the narcotics safe.

9. Turn off the lights.

Note: You may prefer to perform some of these duties in the morning before beginning your day.

Procedure Notes:

6

Aseptic Procedures

Handwashing
What can you do to reduce the spread of pathogens?

Procedure 7-1

Handwashing for Medical Asepsis

1. Assemble this equipment:
   - Liquid soap
   - Paper towels
   - Orangewood stick or nail instrument

2. Remove all rings and wristwatch, or move watch above the wrist several inches.
   Allows proper handwashing procedure; protects items from water damage

3. Stand close to but not touching the sink.
   Prevents splashing; avoids contamination of clothing

4. Turn on the faucet using a paper towel. Discard the towel.
   Prevents contact with contaminated faucets

5. Wet hands and wrists under running warm water and apply liquid antibacterial soap.
   Helps produce lather without drying the integument; helps reduce surface pathogens

6. Work the soap into a lather by rubbing the palms of the hands together, then intertwine the fingers of both hands and rub the soap between the fingers at least 10 times.
   Dislodges microorganisms between fingers

7. Scrub the palm of one hand with the fingertips of the other hand to work the soap under the nails of that hand, then reverse the procedure and scrub the other hand. Scrub the wrists.
Removes microorganisms from nails and wrists

8. Use an orangewood stick under the nails.
Reduces number of microorganisms without causing breaks in protective integumentary barrier

9. Holding the hands in a downward position, rinse the soap from both hands and wrists, allowing the water to drip off the fingertips. Rinse well.
Allows microorganisms to flow off hands and fingers rather than back to arms

10. If hands are grossly contaminated, repeat the procedure.

11. Dry the hands and then the wrists gently with a paper towel. Discard the towel.
Prevents drying and cracking; avoids wicking contaminants back to clean hands

12. Use a dry paper towel to turn off the faucet and discard the towel.
Prevents recontamination

13. If the sink is splattered, wipe with a clean, dry paper towel to remove as many pathogens as possible and to reduce available moisture supportive to growth. Discard the paper towel.

Note: This procedure should take 1 to 2 minutes.

Procedure Notes:

You Need to Know:

- Some facilities have sinks with knee controls, rather than hand controls. Water force is controlled by a back-and-forth motion, and water temperature is controlled by an up-and-down motion. Knee controls are preferred over hand controls for surgical scrubs but may not be available in many office settings. The newest innovation in handwashing uses sensors to activate the water flow and turn it off when the hands are moved beyond the activating device.

Hand Washing for Medical Asepsis

- To avoid chapping and drying your skin with repeated handwashing, use a good-quality lotion between procedures and at night before bed. Breaks in the integument may lead to infection.
- Do not use petroleum-based lotions before gloving; these products cause latex to break down, rendering the protective barrier ineffective.
- Be aware that medical asepsis differs from surgical asepsis (Table 7-1).

Table 7-1

Comparing Medical and Surgical Asepsis

	Medical Asepsis	Surgical Asepsis
Definition	Destroys microorganisms after they leave the body	Destroys microorganisms before they enter the body
Purpose	Prevents the transmission of microorganisms from one person to another	Maintains sterility when entering a normally sterile part of the body
When used	Used when coming in contact with a body part that is not normally sterile (e.g., when performing an enema)	Used when entering a normally sterile part of the body (e.g., when performing urinary catheterization)
Differences in hand-washing technique	Hands and wrists are washed for 1 to 2 minutes; a brush is not necessary. Hands are held down to rinse so that water runs off fingertips. A paper towel is used for drying.	Hands and forearms are washed for 5 to 10 minutes; a brush is used for hands, arms, and nails. Hands are held up to rinse so that water runs off elbows. A sterile towel is used for drying.

Instruct the Patient to:
- Prevent the spread of pathogens by diligent handwashing
- Use and discard paper towels during illness rather than using cloth towels
- Use an antimicrobial soap
- Wash hands before and after meals; after sneezing, coughing, and nose blowing; after using the restroom; before and after procedures requiring contact with blood or body fluid or requiring the use of gloves; and before and after changing a child's diaper.

The surgical scrub reduces surface contaminants to their lowest possible number.

7

Procedure 7-2

Performing a Surgical Scrub

1. Assemble this equipment:
   - Paper towels
   - Liquid antibacterial or bactericidal soap
   - Brush
   - Orangewood stick or nail instrument
   - Sterile towel

2. Remove all jewelry.
   Prevents piercing sterile gloves and contaminating procedure

3. Stand close to but not touching the sink.
   Prevents splashing; avoids contaminating clothing

4. Turn on the faucet using a paper towel. Discard the paper towel.
   Prevents contact with contaminated faucets

5. Wet hands by allowing warm water to flow over them to wet completely. Keep hands above waist level.
   Prevents breaks in integumentary barrier; prevents moisture from returning to washed area

6. Apply liquid bactericidal soap and work into a lather; intertwine the fingers and work the soap between the fingers and around the nails.
   Dislodges microorganisms

7. Using a brush, scrub the nails, backs, and palms of the hands, wrists, and forearms.
   Dislodges and removes the maximum number of microorganisms

BOX 7-1

Standard Precautions

Under Standard Precautions, you must:

- Wash your hands:
  —after touching blood, body fluids, secretions, excretions, and contaminated items, whether you have worn gloves or not
  —immediately after you remove gloves
  —between patient contacts
  —when necessary to prevent transfer of microorganisms
- Use plain soap for routine handwashing and an antimicrobial or antiseptic agent for specified situations.
- Wear clean, nonsterile gloves when touching blood, body fluids, secretions, excretions, mucous membranes, nonintact skin, and contaminated items.
- Change gloves between procedures on the same patient after exposure to potentially infective material.
- Remove gloves immediately after patient contact, and wash your hands.
- Wear protective barrier equipment (e.g., mask, goggles, face shield, gown) to protect the mucous membranes of your eyes, nose, and mouth and to avoid soiling your clothing when performing procedures that may generate splashes or sprays of blood, body fluids, secretions, or excretions.
- Care for equipment and linens that are contaminated with blood, body fluids, secretions, or excretions in a way that avoids skin and mucous membrane exposures, clothing contamination, and microorganism transfer to other patients and environments. Dispose of single-use items appropriately.
- Take precautions to avoid injuries before, during, and after any procedures using needles, scalpels, or other sharp instruments.

Standard Precautions—cont'd

- Ensure that used needles are not recapped, purposely bent, broken, removed from disposable syringes, or otherwise manipulated by hand. Never direct the point of a needle toward any part of your body; instead use a one-handed "scoop" technique or a device designed for holding the needle sheath.

- Place used disposable syringes and needles, used scalpel blades, and all other used sharps in a puncture-resistant container that is located as close to the area of use as possible.

- Use barrier devices (e.g., mouthpieces, resuscitation bags) as alternatives to mouth-to-mouth resuscitation.

Reprinted with permission from "Guidelines for Isolation Precaution in Hospitals" developed by the Centers for Disease Control and Prevention (CDC) and the Hospital Infection Control Practices Advisory Committee (HICPAC), January 1996.

7

8. Using an orangewood stick or nail instrument, clean under each nail.
   Removes microorganisms without injuring the integumentary system

9. Rinse thoroughly.

   a. Rinse from the fingertips to the forearms.

   b. Keep the hands higher than the elbows so that water runs down the arms rather than off of the fingertips.
   Prevents returning microorganisms to cleaned hands

10. Dry from the hands to the forearms with a sterile towel.
    Prevents returning microorganisms to cleaned hands

11. Turn off the faucet with the knee controls or with the elbow, or by using a dry, sterile towel.
    Prevents recontaminating hands

Note: This procedure should take 5 to 10 minutes.

Procedure Notes:

Gloves
Because hands cannot be sterilized, how can you ensure safety during surgical procedures?

Procedure 7-3

Sterile Gloving

1. Assemble this equipment:
   - One packet of proper-sized sterile gloves

2. Follow these Standard Precautions.

3. Remove rings and other jewelry.
   Prevents piercing sterile gloves and contaminating procedure

4. Wash hands using the surgical scrub technique (see previous procedure).
   Reduces microorganisms

5. Place the prepackaged gloves on a clean, dry, flat surface with the cuffed end toward you.

   a. Pull the outer wrapping apart to expose the sterile inner wrapping.

   b. With the cuffs toward you, fold back the inner wrap to expose the gloves.
   Makes proper application easier

6. Grasping the edges of the outer paper, open the package out to its fullest.
   Forms sterile field of inner surface

7. Using your nondominant hand, pick up the dominant-hand glove by grasping the folded edge of the cuff, lifting it up and away from the paper (Figure 7-1). The folded edge of the cuff is contaminated as soon as it is touched with the ungloved hand. Be very careful not to touch the outside surface of the sterile glove with your ungloved hand.
   Prevents contamination of sterile surface

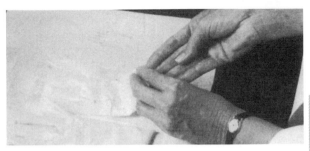

Figure 7-1. Using your nondominant hand, pick up the dominant-hand glove. **7**

8. Curl the fingers and thumb of the dominant hand together to insert them into the glove. Then straighten the fingers and pull the glove on with the nondominant hand still grasping the cuff.
   Prevents accidentally touching outside surface of glove

9. Unfold the cuff by pinching the inside surface that will be against the wrist and pulling it toward the wrist.
   Ensures that only unsterile portions are touched by hands

10. Place the fingers of the gloved hand under the cuff of the remaining glove, lift the glove up and away from the wrapper, and slide the ungloved hand carefully into the glove with the fingers and thumb curled together.
    Avoids sterile glove accidentally touching unsterile surface; ensures that fingers will not brush the sterile surface of glove

11. Straighten the fingers and pull the glove up and over the wrist by carefully unfolding the cuff (Figure 7-2).
    Ensures sterility

12. Settle the gloves comfortably onto the fingers by lacing the fingers together and adjusting the tension over the hands.
    Ensures appropriate fit

Procedure Notes:

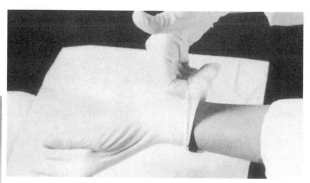

Figure 7-2. Unfold the cuff and pull the glove on snugly.

WARNING!

The incidence of latex allergic reaction is increasing. You or your patient may be sensitive to latex, and your clinical site must provide a suitable alternative. Ask your patient whether a latex allergy exists; if he is unsure, ask whether he has had a reaction to balloons or condoms. It has also been shown that people allergic to bananas, chestnuts, avocados, and several other tropical fruits may be at risk for latex sensitivity. These people are at high risk for a severe reaction if the latex gloves are used on subcutaneous tissues or for extended procedures.

Your gloves are contaminated after use. How should you remove them to protect yourself?

Procedure 7-4

Removing Contaminated Gloves

1. Assemble this equipment:
   • Biohazard container
2. With the gloved dominant hand, grasp the area of glove over the wrist or at the palm of the nondominant hand and pull it away from the hand.
   Avoids touching soiled glove to clean hand

3. Stretch this soiled glove down over your fingers by pulling it away with your gloved hand.
   Frees hand without touching soiled surface

4. As you pull the glove from your hand, ball it into the palm of the still-gloved hand.
   Prevents fingers of glove from accidentally brushing clean area

5. Holding the soiled glove in the palm of the gloved hand, slip your ungloved fingers under the cuff of the gloved hand against the skin, being careful not to touch the soiled outside of the glove (Figure 7-3).
   Avoids contact with soiled area of glove

6. Stretch the glove up and away from your hand, and turn it inside out as it is pulled off over the first glove (Figure 7-4).
   Exposes only clean surfaces; encloses soiled surfaces within gloves

7. Both gloves should now be off, with the first glove inside the palm of the last glove to be removed, and the last glove should be inside out.
   Avoids chance of accidental contamination

8. Discard in a biohazard waste receptacle.

9. Wash your hands well.

Procedure Notes:

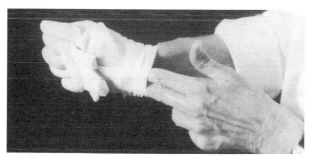

Figure 7-3. Slip your ungloved fingers under the cuff of the gloved hand.

7

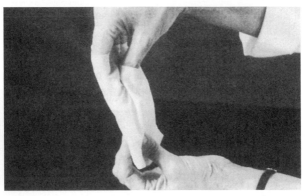

Figure 7-4. Turn the glove inside out as it is pulled over the first glove.

Equipment
How do you prepare equipment and supplies for disinfection or sterilization?

Procedure 7-5

Sanitizing Equipment Before Disinfection or Sterilization

1. Assemble this equipment:
   - Equipment to be sanitized
   - Sanitizing supplies, such as soap, brushes, basins, soaking solutions

2. Follow these Standard Precautions.

       (optional)

3. Choose the appropriate disinfection method (Table 7-2).
   Ensures that items are sanitized properly

4. Take apart pieces that require assembly. If cleaning is not possible immediately, disassemble the pieces and soak the sections to avoid having them stick together.
   Makes cleaning easier and more efficient

Table 7-2

Disinfection Methods

Method	Uses and Precautions
Alcohol (70% isopropyl alcohol or ethyl alcohol)	Used for noncritical items (countertops, oral thermometers, stethoscopes) Flammable Damages some rubber, plastic, and lensed equipment
Chlorine (sodium hypochlorite or bleach)	Dilute to 1:10 (1 part bleach to 10 parts water) Used for a broad spectrum of antimicrobial activity Inexpensive and fast-acting Corrosive, inactivated by organic matter, relatively unstable
Formaldehyde	Disinfectant and sterilant Regulated by Occupational Safety and Health Administration Presence must be marked on all containers and storage areas
Glutaraldehyde	Alkaline or acid-based Effective against bacteria, viruses, fungi, and some spores Regulated by Occupational Safety and Health Administration; requires adequate ventilation, covered pans, gloves, and masks Must display biohazard or chemical label
Hydrogen peroxide	Stable and effective when used on inanimate objects Attacks membrane lipids, DNA, and other essential cell components Can damage plastic, rubber, and some metals
Iodine and iodophores	Bacteriostatic agent used for skin surfaces Not to be used on instruments May cause staining
Phenols (tuberculocidal)	Used for environmental items and equipment Requires gloves and eye protection Can cause skin irritation and burns

5. Check for the operation and integrity of the equipment. If the equipment is defective, it should be repaired or discarded.
Ensures that all items are functional

6. Rinse with cool water.
Prevents sealing proteins onto equipment

7. After the initial rinsing, force streams of soapy water through any tubular or grooved instruments to clean the inside as well as the outside.
Ensures that all surfaces are clean

8. Rinse again in cool water.
Ensures that most proteins are removed from surfaces

9. After the cool rinse, use a hot soapy soak to dissolve fats or lubricants left on the surface. Use the soaking solutions of choice for the facility.
Facilitates cleaning and reduces transient surface microorganisms

10. Use friction with a soft brush or gauze to loosen transient microorganisms. Do not use abrasive materials on delicate instruments and equipment. Brushes work well on grooves and joints. Open and close the jaws of scissors or forceps several times to ensure that all material has been removed.
Ensures that all surfaces are maximally free of microorganisms

11. Rinse well.
Removes soap or detergent residues and remaining microorganisms

12. Dry well before autoclaving or soaking.
Prevents excess moisture that might dilute soaking solution or interfere with proper autoclave procedure

Procedure Notes:

You Need to Know:

• Items used in the sanitation process, such as basins and brushes, are considered grossly contaminated and must be properly sanitized or discarded after use.

After using a glass thermometer, how do you prepare the thermometer for the next patient?

Procedure 7-6

Disinfecting a Glass Thermometer

1. Assemble this equipment:
   - Thermometer to be disinfected
   - Soft tissue or cotton ball
   - Soap

2. Follow these Standard Precautions.

3. Wipe the thermometer with a soft tissue or cotton ball from stem to bulb with a rotating friction.
   Removes most surface substances; prevents returning microorganisms to cleaned area

4. Rub the thermometer briskly with cool or tepid soapy water.
   Prevents damage to the thermometer while allowing effective cleaning

5. Rinse with cool water.
   Removes soapy residue before placing in soaking solution

6. Dry well.
   Prevents diluting soaking solution

7. Place in the disinfectant soaking solution of choice, such as 70% alcohol.
   Prevents heat damage to thermometers; provides appropriate disinfection

8. After the prescribed period of time in the soaking solution of choice, remove the thermometers, rinse them, and store dry.
   Avoids chemical irritation to patient's mucosa

Procedure Notes:

Wrapping Equipment and Supplies for Sterilization

You Need to Know:

- Instructions are provided with the solution that state the time required for disinfection; observe these times carefully.
- Clean and disinfect the soaking basin and storage tray daily using hot soapy water.

How should you wrap instruments to ensure that sterility is maintained?

Procedure 7-7

Wrapping Equipment and Supplies for Sterilization

1. Assemble this equipment:
   - List of items to be included in pack, as needed
   - Sanitized items
   - Sterilization wrap preferred by the facility, appropriate size for items
   - Sterilization indicator
   - Heat-sensitive sealing tape

2. Open all hinged instruments.
   Ensures that steam penetrates all surfaces

3. Place a barrier cloth on the bottom of each tray to be used as a surgical field. If multiple items are to be wrapped together, place the larger, heavier items on the bottom.
   Prevents drips from condensation; protects instruments from damage

4. If sharp-pointed, hinged instruments are to be sterilized, place a cotton ball between the tips before wrapping.
   Prevents piercing the wrap

5. Place the items to be sterilized diagonally on the barrier wrap. If possible or practical, place the items in an order that will facilitate the procedure for which they are prepared.
   a. Fold the closest corner over with a tab folded back.
   b. Fold in the left corner, then fold in the right corner, each with a folded tab.
   c. Fold the last corner over the pack or item and tuck the last corner under the preceding flaps. If the pack is to be double wrapped, follow the same procedure.
   Ensures that items can be unwrapped or opened properly to prevent contamination

6. Seal the items with sterilization indicator tape. Indicate on the tape the contents of the pack, the date of processing, and your initials.
Provides a means of determining that items have been autoclaved, the contents of pack, and the person responsible

Procedure Notes:

You Need to Know:

- If a large surgical setup is processed in a sterilization pouch rather than a wrap, include a drape in the pack to form the sterile field.
- Be aware that site-prepared packs are considered sterile for 30 days.
- When processing single items or small setups in pouches or bags, insert the items so that when the package is opened the instruments will be removed in their functional positions.

What sterilization method is used most often in the medical office?

Procedure 7-8

Operating an Autoclave

1. Assemble this equipment:
  - Sanitized, wrapped articles sealed with indicator tape (packs should contain a sterilization indicator)
  - Distilled water
  - Autoclave operating manual
  - Separately wrapped sterilization indicator

2. Check the autoclave water level and add more if needed, just to the "fill" line.
Provides appropriate quantity of steam for processing

3. Load the autoclave:

  a. Place trays and packs on their sides, from 1 to 3 inches from each other and from the sides of the autoclave.
  Facilitates steam circulation throughout chamber

  b. Put containers on their sides with the lids ajar.
  Allows steam to circulate within containers

7

   c. In mixed loads, place hard objects on the bottom shelf and softer packs on the top racks.
Prevents condensation from hard items from dripping onto softer items

   d. Pack an indicator in the middle of the load.
Provides a means of determining that the procedure was performed properly

4. Read the instructions that should be available near the machine. Almost all machines follow the same protocol:

   a. Close the door and secure it.

   b. Switch on the machine.

   c. When the temperature gauge reaches the temperature required for the contents of the load, usually 250°F or 121°C, set the timer. Many autoclaves can be programmed for the required time.

   d. When the timer indicates that the cycle is over, vent the chamber. Most autoclaves do this automatically.

   e. Be aware that most loads dry in 5 to 20 minutes. Hard items dry faster than soft items.

5. When the load has cooled, remove the items.

6. Check the separately wrapped indicator for proper sterilization.
Verifies that proper autoclave procedure was performed

7. Store the items appropriately in a clean, dry, dust-free area. Site-prepared packs are considered sterile for 30 days.

8. Clean the autoclave per the manufacturer's suggestions, which usually involve scrubbing with a mild detergent and a soft brush. Attention to the exhaust valve prevents lint from occluding the outlet. Rinse the machine thoroughly, and allow it to dry.

Procedure Notes:

Sterile Field
How should you open a sterile pack to ensure sterility?

Procedure 7-9

Preparing a Sterile Field

1. Assemble this equipment:
   - Surgical pack
   - Surgical stand

2. Check the surgical procedure to be performed, and remove the appropriate tray or items from the storage area. Check the label for contents and expiration date. Check for tears or areas of moisture.
   Verifies sterility of package contents

3. Place the package, with the label facing up, on a clean, dry, flat surface, such as a Mayo or surgical stand.
   Provides a convenient area maximally free of microorganisms

4. Without tearing the wrapper, carefully remove the sealing tape. If the package is commercially prepared, carefully remove the outer protective wrapper.
   Avoids contaminating package contents

5. Loosen the first flap of the folded wrapper. Open the first flap by pulling it up, out, and away; let it fall over the far side of the table.
   Prevents reaching over the sterile field

6. Open the side flaps in a similar manner using the left hand for the left flap, right hand for right flap (Figure 7-5). Touch only the unsterile outer surface; do not touch the sterile inner surface.
   Decreases movement over sterile areas of package

7. Pull the remaining flap down and toward you by grasping the unsterile outside surface only. The unsterile surface of the wrapper is now against the surgical stand; the sterile inside surface of the wrapper forms the sterile field.

8. Repeat steps 4 through 7 for packages with a second or inside wrapper. This sterile wrapper also provides a sterile field on which to work. The field is now ready for additional supplies as needed or for the procedure to begin.

Preparing a Sterile Field

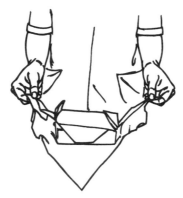

Figure 7-5. Open the side flaps.

Procedure Notes:

WARNING!

If you suspect that the field has been contaminated, you must view the field as nonsterile and begin the procedure again with new, sterile supplies and equipment. Sterility must be reestablished before the procedure can continue.

You Need to Know:

- Do not let sterile packages become damp or wet. Water containing microorganisms may be wicked to the sterile surfaces, and this requires that the package be reprocessed. If liquids are spilled onto the field, the field is considered contaminated.
- Always face the sterile field. If it is necessary to work with your back to the field or to leave the area after opening the field, cover the tray and its contents with a sterile drape.
- Hold sterile items above waist level to avoid inadvertent contamination. A 1-inch border around a sterile field is considered contaminated. Keep sterile items in the middle of the field.
- To avoid contaminating the field, do not cough, sneeze, talk, laugh, or reach across the field.
- Provide a basin on the side to receive used equipment and supplies. These should not be returned to the field.

- At the completion of the procedure, discard any commercially wrapped items that were not used for the sterile procedure for which they were opened.

Follow these steps when sterile solutions must be added to the field.

Procedure 7-10

Adding a Sterile Solution to the Sterile Field

1. Assemble this equipment:
   - Container of sterile solution
   - Sterile setup

2. As with any drug or medication, identify the correct solution by carefully reading the label three times.

3. Check for an expiration date on the label; do not use the solution if it is out of date, if the label cannot be read, or if the solution appears abnormal.
   Ensures that solution is current and correct

4. If you are adding medications to the solution (e.g., lidocaine, a local anesthetic), show the medication label to the physician now.
   Allows verification of contents

5. With sterile transfer forceps, move any solution receptacles close to the edge of the sterile field, but well within the 1-inch border.
   Prevents reaching across the sterile field

6. Remove the cap or stopper. Hold the cap with the finger tips, with the cap opening facing downward, to prevent accidental contamination of the inside. If it is necessary to put the cap down, place it with the opened end facing up. If you are pouring the entire contents of the container onto the sterile field, discard the cap. (Retain the bottle to keep track of the amount added to the field and for charting purposes later. It can then be discarded.)
   Prevents contaminating the cap and contents

7. Grasp the container so that the label is facing the palm of the hand, that is, "palm the label."
   Prevents obscuring the label if solution runs down the side of the bottle

8. Pour a small amount of the solution into a separate container or waste receptacle.

Cleanses bottle lip

9. Carefully and slowly pour the desired amount of solution into the sterile container from not less than 4 inches and not more than 6 inches above the container. The bottle of solution should never touch the sterile container or tray because this will cause contamination.

Reduces splashing or overfilling; prevents touching the field

10. After pouring the desired amount of solution into the sterile container, recheck the label for contents and expiration date, and replace the cap carefully to avoid touching the bottle rim with any unsterile surface of the cap.

Ensures accuracy; maintains sterility of contents

11. Return the solution to its proper storage area, and check the label again.

Ensures accuracy

Procedure Notes:

You Need to Know:

• Sterile water and saline bottles must be dated when opened and must be discarded if not used within 48 hours. Out-of-date solutions may have changed chemically or deteriorated, and are no longer considered sterile.

How can you safely add supplies to a sterile field or move them within the field?

Procedure 7-11

Using Sterile Transfer Forceps

1. Assemble this equipment:
   • Forceps and container
   • Items to be transferred

2. Slowly lift the forceps straight up and out of the container without touching the inside above the level of the solution or the outside of the container.
Prevents touching contaminated areas

3. Hold the forceps with the tips down.
Avoids returning solution to unsterile handles and back to grasping blades and tips

4. Keep the forceps above waist level.
Prevents accidental and unnoticed contamination

5. Pick up the article to be transferred, and drop it into the sterile field so that the forceps do not come in contact with the sterile field.
Avoids contact between moist forceps and sterile field

Procedure Notes:

You Need to Know:

- Place sterile transfer forceps that have been wrapped and autoclaved with the tips on the sterile field and with handles extending beyond the 1-inch contaminated perimeter. You may grasp the handles that extend beyond the perimeter if you need to move objects around the field for the physician's convenience.
- In a closed, dry container, autoclave the forceps and container daily. In a closed, sterile solution system, resterilize both the forceps and container daily, and add fresh solution.
- Store only one set of forceps per container to avoid tangling or contamination.

What should you do if hazardous material spills?

Procedure 7-12

Cleaning and Decontaminating Biohazardous Spills

1. Assemble this equipment:
 · Disposable towels or other absorbent material
 · Germicide, such as 1:10 chlorine bleach

2. Follow these Standard Precautions.

3. Wear protective eyewear and an impervious gown if splashing may occur.
Protects against exposure to hazardous material

4. Remove visible material with disposable towels or other means that prevent contact with the fluid.
Reduces the quantity of surface contaminants

5. Dispose of the material in a biohazard container.
Protects against accidental exposure

6. Decontaminate the area with an appropriate germicide, and discard the material used for wiping up the area in an appropriate biohazard container.
Secures area and contaminated material for disposal

7. Place all soiled items in the biohazard container, and dispose of the container and items according to facility policy. Biohazard bags should be available for removal of contaminated items from the site of the spill.
Ensures appropriate disposal of biohazardous waste

8. Wash your hands after removing and discarding the gloves.

Procedure Notes:

You Need to Know:

- Before using any disinfecting products, read the Material Safety Data Sheets (MSDS) for proper handling and disposal of chemicals.

WARNING!

Your shoes can become contaminated with biohazardous material as well. Where there is massive contamination on floors, consider using disposable impervious shoe coverings. Wear protective gloves to remove contaminated shoe coverings. Dispose of the gloves and coverings in biohazard containers.

8

Assessment Procedures

Diagnosing existing conditions requires a strong medical history.

Procedure 8-1

Interviewing the Patient to Obtain a Medical History

1. Assemble this equipment:
   - Medical history form or questionnaire
   - Any available previous patient information
   - Pen

2. Follow these Standard Precautions.

3. Review the medical history form.
   Enhances familiarity with order of questions and type of information required

4. Find a private and comfortable place.
   Avoids distractions and ensures confidentiality

5. Sit across from the patient at eye level and maintain frequent eye contact.
   Increases rapport and facilitates communication

6. Introduce yourself and explain the purpose of the interview.
   Establishes professional rapport with patient

Interviewing the Patient to Obtain a Medical History

7. Using language the patient can understand, ask the appropriate questions and document the patient's responses. Be sure to determine the patient's chief complaint (CC) and present illness (PI).
   Assists in obtaining accurate and complete data

8. Listen actively, stop writing from time to time, and look at the patient while he or she is speaking.
   Encourages cooperation

9. Regardless of the confidences shared by the patient, avoid projecting a judgmental attitude by your words or your actions.
   Maintains professionalism and ensures the patient's trust

10. If appropriate, explain to the patient what to expect during any examination or procedures that may be scheduled for the day.
    Keeps patient informed regarding his or her care

11. Thank the patient for cooperating during the interview, and offer to answer any questions.
    Encourages a positive attitude about the office and physician

Procedure Notes:

You Need to Know:

- Barriers to communication may interfere with eliciting an adequate patient history. Review your textbook regarding methods for overcoming common barriers. If the communication barrier is language-based, refer to a translation list of English to the appropriate language, and keep a good reference manual nearby. Learn as many phrases in your local second language as possible.

Instruct the Patient to:

- Bring a list of questions with each visit, to increase a feeling of participation in health care
- Compile a list or bring all medications, prescribed or over-the-counter, at each visit

Document on the Patient's Chart:

* Date and time
* Height and weight
* Vital signs as required by office protocol
* All laboratory values obtained as required by office protocol
* Patient complaints or concerns
* Patient education and instructions
* Your signature

EXAMPLE

8

1/14/2004	CC: Physical exam for employment.
10:45 AM	Ht. 6'1" Wt. 178# T: 98.8 (o), P: 84
	reg, R: 16, BP 128/78 (L). Urinalysis:
	pH 6.5 sp grav 1.020 ketones, blood,
	protein, glucose neg. Visual acuity
	20/20 OU without correction.
	—J. Brown CMA

Is your patient's weight appropriate for his or her height?

Procedure 8-2

Measuring Height

1. Assemble this equipment:
   * Scale with ruler or standard marked or mounted on the wall
2. Follow these Standard Precautions.

3. Have the patient stand straight and erect on the scale, heels together, eyes straight ahead. If measurement is against the wall standard, the posture requirements are the same.
Ensures accurate measurement

4. With the measurement bar perpendicular to the ruler, slowly lower it until it touches the patient's head. Press lightly if the hair is full and high.
Measures height, not hair

5. Read the measurement at the point of movement on the ruler. If the measurements are in inches (with smaller marks for $\frac{1}{4}$, $\frac{1}{2}$, $\frac{3}{4}$), convert the inches to feet and inches. Example: If the point of movement reads 65 plus two smaller lines, read it as $65\frac{1}{2}$. Remember that 12 inches equals 1 foot; therefore, the patient is 5 feet $5\frac{1}{2}$ inches tall.

6. At the completion of the procedure, assist the patient from the scale.
Ensures patient safety

7. Record the patient's height. If this measurement is recorded on a graph, carefully align the point to accurately reflect the patient's measurement.

8. Return the measure bar to a safe position for the next procedure.

Procedure Notes:

You Need to Know:

- If the physician prefers inches to centimeters or vice versa, the ruler provided should be in the preferred measurement. If it is necessary to convert from inches to centimeters or vice versa, remember that 1 inch = 2.5 cm.

  —To convert inches to centimeters, multiply the number of inches by 2.5.
  —To convert centimeters to inches, divide the number of centimeters by 2.5.

Document on the Patient's Chart:

- Date and time
- Patient's height in preferred measurement
- Patient complaints or concerns
- Your signature

EXAMPLE

9/15/2004	CC: c/o increased cervicothoracic
10:15 AM	spinal curvature and pain due to
	"arthritis," Ht. 5'2 1/2" Wt. 125#
	T 98.6 (o) P 88 reg R 20 BP
	134/84 (R). Currently taking OTC
	meds (ibuprofen) for pain relief.
	Ht. x5 yrs. ago 5'4".
	—L. Burroughs CMA

8

A comparison between height and weight helps assess the patient's health and nutritional status.

Procedure 8-3

Measuring Weight

1. Assemble this equipment:
   - Calibrated scale
   - Paper towel

2. Follow these Standard Precautions.

3. Ensure that the scale is properly calibrated by observing that the balance beam hangs freely at the midpoint when the counterweights are resting at zero.
Avoids errors in measurement

4. Greet and identify the patient. Explain the procedure.

5. Escort the patient to the scale. Place a paper towel on the scale.
Minimizes microorganism transmission; increases patient comfort

6. Make sure the scale is balanced at zero.
Eliminates one source of possible error

7. Have the patient remove shoes and heavy coat or jacket, put down purse, and step up onto the scale.
Ensures accurate measurement

8. Assist the patient onto the scale. Have the patient stand steady without touching anything; watch closely for loss of balance.
Increases patient safety

9. Weigh the patient.

    a. On a balance beam scale: Slide the counterweights on the bottom and top bars from zero to the approximate weight, and then adjust to the proper weight. Each counterweight should rest securely in its notch, with the indicator mark at the proper calibration. To obtain the measurement, the balance bar must hang freely at the exact midpoint. To calculate the weight, add the top reading to the bottom reading. Example: If the bottom counterweight reads 100 and the top one reads 16 plus three small lines, the weight is $116\frac{3}{4}$ lb.

    b. On a digital scale: Read the weight, which is displayed automatically on the digital screen.

    c. On a dial scale: The indicator arrow rests at the proper weight. Read this number from directly above the dial.
Prevents errors in measurement

Procedure Notes:

Document on the Patient's Chart:

- Date and time
- Patient's weight, indicated in pounds or kilograms
- Any patient data regarding weight progression or diet
- Patient complaints or concerns
- Patient education and instructions
- Your signature

EXAMPLE

3/6/2004	CC: Return for weight check. Wt.: 230 lb
3:30 PM	T 97.8 (o) P 96 reg R 24 BP 166/86
	(L). Wt. at last visit 233#. Pt. has no
	complaints, states he is adhering to
	prescribed diet, has appointment with
	dietitian in 10 days.
	—K. Morgan CMA

8

You Need to Know:

- If the physician prefers pounds to kilograms or vice versa, the preferred scale will usually be provided. If it is necessary to convert pounds to kilograms or vice versa, remember that 1 kg = 2.2 lb.

  —To change pounds to kilograms, divide the number of pounds by 2.2.

  —To change kilograms to pounds, multiply the number of kilograms by 2.2.

- Certain circumstances require that the patient be weighed wearing only a gown. In this situation, ensure patient privacy by moving the scale to the examining room where the gowned patient is waiting.

- Many patients are uncomfortable with their weight. Do not announce the patient's weight in an exposed area. In the privacy of the examination room, ask the patient if he or she would like to know the reading.

Performing a 12-Lead Electrocardiogram

- Speak with his or her physician regarding a proper diet or a referral to a registered dietitian or nutritionist for weight management

What is the single most useful noninvasive cardiac procedure for diagnosing cardiac arrhythmias?

Procedure 8-4

Performing a 12-Lead Electrocardiogram

1. Assemble this equipment:
   - Electrocardiogram (ECG) machine with cable and lead wires
   - ECG paper if not part of machine
   - Disposable electrodes that contain coupling gel
   - Gown or cape and drape
   - Skin preparation materials, including razor and antiseptic wipes

2. Follow these Standard Precautions.

3. Greet and identify the patient. Explain the procedure, noting that the machine picks up tremors or muscle movement and instructing the patient to lie still for the usually brief duration of the test. Ask for and answer any questions.

4. Turn the machine on and enter appropriate data into the ECG machine, including the patient's name and/or identification number, age, sex, height, weight, and medications.
   This information will be printed on the ECG printout and will assist the physician in determining a proper diagnosis.

5. Instruct the patient to disrobe above the waist, and provide a gown for privacy. Female patients should also be instructed to remove any nylons or tights.
   Clothing may interfere with proper lead placement.

8

6. Position the patient comfortably in a supine position with pillows as needed for comfort. Drape the patient for warmth and privacy.

If the patient is uncomfortable, too cool, or improperly draped, movement is likely, which will result in artifact on the ECG tracing.

7. Prepare the skin as needed by wiping away skin oil and lotions with the antiseptic wipes or by shaving any excess hair.

Skin preparation ensures properly attached leads and helps avoid improper readings and time lost in repeating the procedure.

8. Apply the electrodes snugly against the fleshy, muscular parts of the upper arms and lower legs according to the manufacturer's directions (Figure 8-1).

Electrodes that are not snug against the skin or that are placed on bony prominences may cause an improper reading and artifact.

9. Connect the lead wires securely according to the color-coded notations on the connectors (RA, LA, RL, LL, V1-V6). Untangle the wires before applying to decrease electrical artifacts. Each lead must lie unencumbered along the contours of the patient's body to decrease the incidence of artifacts. Double-check the placement.

Improperly placed leads will result in time lost due to an inaccurate reading and to retesting.

10. Determine the sensitivity or gain and paper speed settings on the ECG machine before running the 12-lead ECG. The sensitivity or gain should be set on "1" and the paper speed should be set on 25 mm/sec.

A sensitivity or gain setting of "1" and a paper speed of 25 mm/sec are necessary for obtaining an accurate ECG; these settings should not be changed without a direct order from the physician, and if changes are made, these should be noted on the final ECG tracing.

11. Depress the automatic button on the ECG machine to obtain the 12-lead ECG tracing. The machine will automatically move from one lead to the next without intervention from the medical assistant.

If the physician only wants a rhythm strip tracing, the manual mode of operation will need to be used and the lead desired will be selected manually.

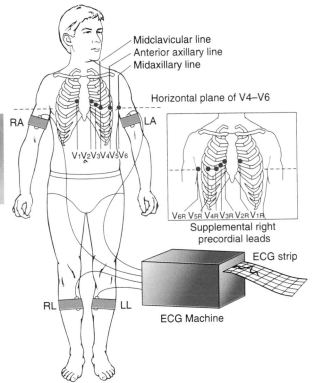

Figure 8-1. Twelve-lead ECG electrode placement.

12. When the tracing is complete and printed, check the
ECG for artifact and a standardization mark.

*With the machine sensitivity set on "1," the standardization mark
should be 2 small squares wide and 10 small squares high. The
standardization mark documents accuracy of operation and provides a reference point. Tracings with artifact will need to have the
source of the artifact corrected and the tracing redone.*

13. If the tracing is adequate, turn the machine off and remove the electrodes from the patient's skin. Assist the
patient to a sitting position and help with dressing if
needed. Some patients may become dizzy from lying
supine.

14. If a single-channel machine was used (each lead is produced on a roll of paper, one lead at a time), carefully roll the ECG strip without using clips to secure the roll. This ECG will need to be mounted on a special form to be placed into the patient's medical record (Table 8-1).
Folding the ECG tracing or applying clips may make marks on the surface of the ECG, obscuring the tracing and making interpretation difficult.

15. Record the procedure in the patient's medical record.
Procedures are considered not to have been done if they are not recorded.

16. Place the ECG tracing and the patient's medical record on the physician's desk or give to the physician for diagnosis and interpretation.

Procedure Notes:

You Need to Know:

- If the patient is suspected of having had a MI (complaints of chest pain, pressure), the physician may want to check the ECG strip before the electrodes are removed to avoid having to replace them for a repeat ECG.
- ECG lead placement is designed to provide the most diagnostic evaluation; however, it may be necessary to alter the placement on certain patients, including amputees and postoperative limb surgery patients. Note the lead placement in the patient record and on the

Table 8-1

Coding ECG Leads

Lead	Code	Lead	Code
I	.	V1	-.
II	..	V2	-..
III	...	V3	-...
aVR	-	V4	-....
aVL	--	V5	-.....
aVF	---	V6	-......

Document on the Patient's Chart:

- Date and time
- Performance of procedure
- Ordering physician or physician evaluating the reading
- Patient complaints or concerns
- Patient education and instructions
- Your signature

EXAMPLE

9/8/2004	12-lead ECG done and given to Dr. Bruno
3:30 PM	for evaluation. Denied c/o of chest pain
	before and during the procedure.
	—A. Perez, CMA

database section of the mounting device if other than the standard placement is used.
- Keep the patient warm and comfortable enough to prevent movement and shivering to avoid somatic tremors.

Instruct the Patient to:

- Lie still to avoid having to repeat the procedure because of somatic artifacts

Is your patient's arrhythmia intermittent in nature? The Holter monitor is the test of choice.

Procedure 8-5

Applying a Holter Monitor

1. Assemble this equipment:
   - Monitor
   - Fresh batteries
   - Roll of blank tape
   - Carrying case with strap
   - Electrodes
   - Skin swabs
   - Gauze

- Razor, as needed
- Patient diary

2. Follow these Standard Precautions.

  (optional)

3. Greet and identify the patient. Explain the procedure. Remind the patient that it is important to carry out all normal activities for the duration of the test.

4. Explain the purpose for the incident diary, emphasizing the need for the patient to carry it at all times during the test.

5. Prepare the patient's skin for electrode attachment. Provide privacy and have the patient sit. Expose the chest, then shave the areas of attachment as needed. Glove if shaving is required. Clean with the approved defatting agent to remove skin oils. Abrade the area with the gauze.
Ensures proper placement of electrodes; improves skin adherence of electrode adhesive

6. Apply the special Holter electrodes at the specified sites (Figure 8-2). To do this, expose the adhesive backing of the electrodes and follow manufacturer's instructions to attach firmly. Check for security of attachment. The sites are:

   a. The right manubrium border

   b. The left manubrium border

   c. The right sternal border at the fifth rib level

   d. The fifth rib at the anterior axillary line

   e. The right lower rib cage over the cartilage as a ground lead
   Ensures proper placement; provides secure adhesion for duration of testing

7. Position electrode connectors pointing downward toward the patient's feet. Attach the leads and secure with adhesive tape.
Secures leads

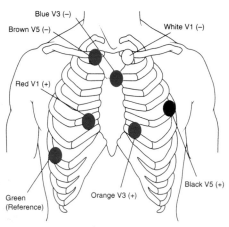

Brown V5 (–)
Blue V3 (–)
White V1 (–)
Red V1 (+)
Green (Reference)
Orange V3 (+)
Black V5 (+)

Figure 8-2. Sites for Holter monitor electrodes.

8. Connect the cable and run a baseline ECG by hooking the Holter to the ECG machine with the cable hookup.
Confirms accurate function of monitor

9. Assist the patient to redress carefully with the cable extending through a garment opening. Clothing that buttons down the front is more convenient.
Prevents tension on leads

10. Plug the cable into the recorder and mark the diary. Review the purpose of the diary with the patient again. Schedule a return appointment.

Procedure Notes:

You Need to Know:

- Fresh batteries preclude battery failure, and a whole roll of monitor tape prevents the patient from running out of tape during the test.
- Lead placement also may include electrodes at the left manubrium border at the second rib and the left sternal border at the fifth intercostal space.

Document on the Patient's Chart:

- Date and time
- Application of monitor
- Patient education and instructions
- Date and time scheduled for return
- Your signature

EXAMPLE

11/28/2004	Holter monitor applied as ordered—
2:00 PM	baseline ECG done. Verbal and written
	instructions given regarding the care
	of the monitor and electrodes and the
	completion of the diary. Pt. instructed
	to RTO tomorrow for removal. Pt. ver-
	balized understanding.
	—K. Steele, CMA

8

Instruct the Patient to:

- Maintain a normal routine during monitoring to provide an accurate evaluation of cardiac stress factors

Evaluating the ECG reading is easier for the physician when it is properly mounted for interpretation.

Procedure 8-6

Mounting the ECG Strip for Evaluation

1. Assemble this equipment:
   - Physician-preferred mounting device
   - Clean, flat surface
   - Scissors

2. Follow these Standard Precautions.

3. Label the mounting paper with the patient's data.
Provides information for interpretation of strip

4. Unroll the strip on a clean, flat surface, and identify the area of Lead 1 with the standardization mark. Cut this strip with scissors to the length preferred by the physician.
Provides standardization mark for reference

5. If the mounting device has protective sleeves, carefully open the sleeve as far as possible and insert the strip. If the mounting papers have adhesive strips and clear plastic covers, use care to prevent marring the surface of the strip.
Prevents obscuring strip

6. Repeat the procedure until all of the leads are in their proper places on the sheet.

7. File the report in the area the physician has designated for reports pending review.

Procedure Notes:

You Need to Know:

• Physicians have individual preferences regarding the proper length for various types of readings; determine the length preferred by the evaluating physician before cutting the strips.

What can you do to help your patient and physician during the physical examination?

Procedure 8-7

Assisting With the Physical Examination

1. Assemble this equipment:
• Appropriate instruments may include stethoscope, ophthalmoscope, penlight, otoscope, tuning fork, nasal speculum, tongue blade, laryngeal mirror, percussion hammer, vaginal speculum

- Glass of water (optional)
- Substances for testing sense of smell (optional)
- Gauze squares
- Lubricant
- Vaginal spatula or histobrush
- Slides, slide covers, and fixative
- Requisition slips, as appropriate
- Tissues
- Specimen container
- Gown
- Drape
- Electrocardiograph

8

2. Follow these Standard Precautions.

3. Prepare the examining room.
   Prevents transfer of microorganisms; ensures that all equipment is functional and available

4. Greet the patient by name and escort to the examining room.

5. Explain the procedures.

6. Obtain and record the medical history and chief complaint, if that is your responsibility.
   Gives background information about health and symptoms

7. Obtain and record the patient's temperature, pulse, respiration rate, blood pressure, height, and weight, and check for visual acuity. Draw blood if necessary for testing and route as needed.
   Gives overall picture of current health

8. Instruct the patient in obtaining a urine specimen and escort him or her to the restroom.
   Provides data on general health; facilitates palpation of abdomen

9. See that the specimen is properly labeled and received in the laboratory.

10. Escort the patient back to the examining room. Instruct the patient to disrobe completely and put on a

gown opening down the back or front as directed by the physician. Leave the room unless the patient needs assistance.

Provides accessibility for examination; provides privacy or assistance as needed

11. Perform an electrocardiogram if ordered.

Provides information regarding heart's conduction system

12. Assist the patient into a sitting position on the edge of the examination table (Figure 8-3). Cover the lap and legs with a drape sheet.

Ensures patient is in correct position for examination; provides privacy

8

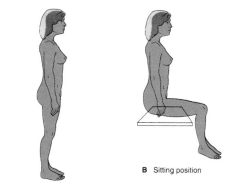

B Sitting position

A Erect or standing position

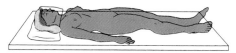

C Supine position

Figure 8-3. Patient examination positions. (A) Standing position. The patient's body is erect and facing forward with the arms down at the sides. (B) Sitting position. The patient sits erect at the end of the examination table with the feet supported. (C) Supine position. The patient lies on the back with the arms at the side. A pillow is usually placed under the head for comfort.

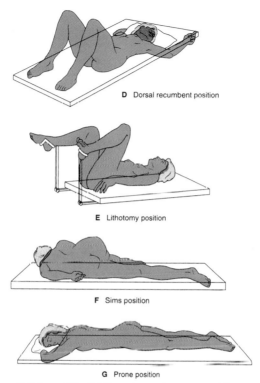

D Dorsal recumbent position

E Lithotomy position

F Sims position

G Prone position

Figure 8-3 (cont'd). (D) Dorsal recumbent position. The patient is in the supine position with the legs separated, knees bent, and feet flat on the table. (E) Lithotomy position. The position is similar to the dorsal recumbent position, but the patient's feet are placed in stirrups rather than flat on the table. The stirrups should be level with each other and about one foot from the edge of the table. The patient's legs should be moved simultaneously to prevent back strain. (F) Sims position. The patient lies on the left side with the left arm and shoulder behind the body, the right leg and arm sharply flexed on the table, and the left knee slightly flexed. (G) Prone position. The patient lies on the abdomen with the head supported and turned to one side. The arms may be placed under the head or by the sides, whichever is more comfortable.

continued

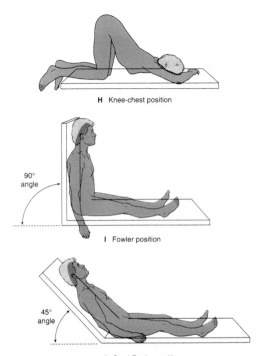

H Knee-chest position

I Fowler position

90° angle

45° angle

J Semi-Fowler position

Figure 8-3 (cont'd). (H) Knee-chest position. The patient kneels on the table with the arms and chest on the table, hips in the air, and back straight. (I) Fowler position. The patient is in a semi-sitting position with the head of the bed elevated 80° to 90°. (J) Semi-Fowler position. The patient is in a semi-sitting position with the head of the bed elevated 30° to 45° and the knees slightly bent.

13. Place the patient's chart outside the examination room door, and notify the physician that the patient is ready.
Prevents delays

14. Assist the physician during the examination by handing the instruments needed for examination of each body area and ensuring proper patient positioning.

   a. Begin by handing the physician the instrument necessary for examination:
   - Head and neck: stethoscope and glass of water
   - Eyes: ophthalmoscope, penlight
   - Ears: otoscope, tuning fork
   - Nose: nasal speculum, penlight, substances for testing sense of smell
   - Sinuses: penlight
   - Mouth: glove, gauze square, tongue blade, penlight
   - Throat: glove, tongue blade, laryngeal mirror, penlight

   Promotes efficiency and saves time

   b. Assist the patient in removing the gown to the waist so the physician can examine the chest and upper back. Hand the physician the stethoscope to assess sounds within the thorax.

   Exposes only parts being examined

   c. Assist the patient in putting on the gown, and remove the drape sheet from the legs so that the physician may test the reflexes. Hand the physician the reflex hammer

   d. Assist the patient to a supine position, opening the gown at the top to expose the chest once again. Place the drape sheet from the waist down to the toes. Hand the physician the stethoscope to assess cardiac sounds.

8

e. Cover the patient's chest and lower the drape sheet to the pubic area to expose the abdomen. The physician uses the stethoscope to assess bowel sounds.

f. Assist with genital and rectal examinations. Hand the patient tissues following these examinations.
Wipes away excess lubricant

For Female Patients:
- Assist the patient into the lithotomy position and drape appropriately.
- For examination of the genitalia and internal reproductive organs, provide a glove, lubricant, speculum, spatula or brush, slides, fixative, slide covers, and requisition slip.
- For rectal examination, provide a glove, lubricant, slides, slide covers, and requisition slip.

For Male Patients:
- Assist the patient to a standing position. In this position, the physician can check for a hernia; by having the patient bend over the table, the physician can perform a rectal and prostate examination.
- For hernia examination, provide a glove.
- For rectal examination, provide a glove, lubricant, slide covers, and requisition slip.
- For prostate examination, provide a glove and lubricant.

15. Help the patient to return to a sitting position at the edge of the examining table.
Allows opportunity for physician to discuss examination findings and provide instruction

16. Perform any follow-up procedures or treatments.
Ensures that no health care directives are omitted

17. Leave the room while the patient dresses unless needed for assistance with clothing.
Provides privacy

18. Return to the room to answer questions, reinforce instructions, and provide patient education.
Reinforces compliance and understanding

19. Escort the patient to the front office.
Provides an opportunity to clarify appointment scheduling or billing questions

20. Properly clean or dispose of all used equipment. Clean the room with disinfectant and prepare for the next patient. Wash your hands.

Procedure Notes:

8

You Need to Know:

- Patients with special needs may require a longer examination time than other patients; ensure that adequate time is set aside for special assistance and for questions. Read your reference sources for barriers to communication for helpful suggestions, as needed.
- Occasionally, patients who do not need assistance before the examination may need help at its completion. Do not leave the patient alone until you have determined whether your assistance is needed.
- During the examination, hand the tongue blade to the physician by holding it in the middle. When it is returned to you after use, grasp it in the middle again so that you do not touch the end that was in the patient's mouth. Warm the laryngeal mirror in warm water to prevent fogging.

Instruct the Patient or Caregiver to:

- Compile a list of questions for each visit so that no concerns are forgotten
- Ask questions brought up by the examination
- Call back if questions occur after the examination

Document on the Patient's Chart:
- Date and time
- Patient complaints or concerns
- Anthropometric measurements and vital signs as required by office protocol
- Results of routine office laboratory procedures
- Special preparations or procedures for the examination
- Patient education and instructions
- Your signature

8

EXAMPLE

4/15/2004	CC: 45-year-old male, initial physical
1:00 PM	exam. Ht. 5'7" Wt. 138# T 98.2 tym-
	panic P 92 reg, R 14 BP 122/76 (R).
	Medical history form completed with
	minimal assistance. Pt. given new pa-
	tient brochure.
	—Y. Torres, CMA

Need to provide the physician with the diagnostic set for examination of the eye and ear? Use the following guides.

Procedure 8-8

Preparing the Diagnostic Set

1. Assemble this equipment:
   - Otoscope
   - Ophthalmoscope
   - Tongue blade holder (optional)
   - Power source, such as an electrical charger or fresh battery

2. Follow these Standard Precautions.

3. Check to determine that the lights in the instrument are functioning by illuminating them.
Establishes function before procedure

4. Check the otoscope, ophthalmoscope, and illuminated tongue blade holder for function. Press firmly and twist to place or remove the head. The small red button at the connection is held down as the rim is rotated to keep the light on. Reverse the procedure to turn it off.
Verifies function of each item

8

5. Place tongue blades and disposable ear specula on a covered tray for the physician's use.
Provides easy access to items

6. Have extra light bulbs available for replacement during the examination, if needed.
Ensures availability of light source

Procedure Notes:

Can a patient perceive color? The Ishihara test determines deficits in color perception.

Procedure 8-9

Measuring Color Perception

1. Assemble this equipment:
 • Ishihara color plates
 • Gloves

2. Follow these Standard Precautions.

3. Put on gloves.
Prevents damage to color plates from oils on hands

Document on the Patient's Chart:

- Date and time
- Observations of the patient during testing
- Results of testing
- Your signature

EXAMPLE

3/2/2004	Color perception assessed using
11:20 AM	Ishihara plates. Pt. successfully
	identified all plates except #9—Dr.
	Barker notified.
	—J. Crosby

4. Identify the patient and explain the procedure for the first plate. Hold the plate about 30 inches from the patient.
Serves as example for following plates

5. Ensure that the patient is in a comfortable sitting position in a quiet, well-lighted room. Indirect sunlight gives the best illumination.
Provides adequate light for testing; protects chart from damage from direct sunlight

6. Follow directions on the chart to test the patient's right eye, then the left eye.

7. Thank the patient and give appropriate instructions.

Procedure Notes:

<hr>

You Need to Know:

- Record the results of the test by noting what the patient reports seeing on each plate that is read incorrectly, using the plate number and the answer given by the patient. If the patient cannot distinguish any pattern, record as "Plate no. 3 = X." It is not necessary to record those plates read correctly.

- Record any squinting, tearing, or any hesitation or guesses indicating that the patient is not sure of what is being perceived.
- Store the book in a closed, protected area to protect the integrity of the colors.
- Patients who wear glasses or contact lenses may keep them on. The Ishihara method tests color acuity, not visual acuity. Corrective lenses do not interfere with accurate test results.

How would you test a patient's ability to focus on far objects?

Procedure 8-10

Measuring Distant Visual Acuity   8

1. Assemble this equipment:
  - Eye chart
  - Paper cup or eye paddle

2. Follow these Standard Precautions.

3. Prepare the examination room. Make sure the area is well lighted. A mark should indicate the distance 20 feet from the chart; the chart must be at eye level.
Helps elicit best response; standard distance provides consistency of results

4. Greet and identify the patient. Explain the procedure.

5. Position the patient in a standing or sitting position at the 20-foot marker.

6. Ask if the patient wears glasses or contact lenses. Mark the record accordingly.
Provides accurate documentation

7. Have the patient cover the left eye with the eye paddle. Instruct the patient to keep both eyes open.
Complies with routine testing measures

8. Stand beside the chart and point to each row as the patient reads aloud the indicated lines, starting with the 20/200 line.
Ensures that patient is reading the correct line; starts with line easiest to read

8

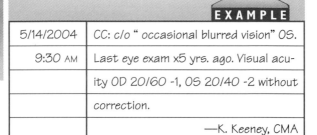

Document on the Patient's Chart:
- Date and time
- Patient complaints or concerns
- Observations of patient during test, including with or without corrective lenses
- Test results: OD, OS, OU (oculi unitas)
- Your signature

EXAMPLE

5/14/2004	CC: c/o " occasional blurred vision" OS.
9:30 AM	Last eye exam x5 yrs. ago. Visual acu-
	ity OD 20/60 -1, OS 20/40 -2 without
	correction.
	—K. Keeney, CMA

9. Record the smallest line the patient can read without error and note as OD (oculus dexter). The numbers are listed on the side of the chart. For instance, if the patient reads line five or the line marked 40 with one error for the right eye, record as OD 20/40-1. Your physician may prefer that only those lines read without error be counted as correct.

10. Repeat the procedure with the right eye covered and record as in step 9, using OS (oculus sinister).

11. Thank the patient and give appropriate instructions.

12. Wash your hands.

Procedure Notes:

You Need to Know:
- The patient may stand or sit, if necessary, as long as the chart is at eye level and the patent is 20 feet from the chart.
- Office policy states whether examinations may include corrective lenses. The patient record should indicate whether the patient wears corrective lenses for the test.

- The hand may not be used to cover the eye to avoid pressure against the eye or peeking through the fingers.
- It is generally best to start at about the second or third row to judge the patient's response. If these lines are read easily, move down to smaller figures. If the patient has trouble reading the larger lines, notify the physician.
- If the patient squints or leans forward, record this observation on the patient record. Squinting to close one eye changes the visual perception.

Use this test if a patient complains that he can no longer see small print.

Procedure 8-11

8

Measuring Near Visual Acuity

1. Assemble this equipment:
   - Jaegar near visual acuity testing card
   - Paper cup or eye paddle

2. Follow these Standard Precautions.

3. Greet and identify the patient. Explain the procedure. Ask for and answer any questions.

4. Hold the card containing lines of text or pictures of Es to be evaluated about 14 to 16 inches from the patient's face at a comfortable reading level.
   Provides normal reading distance for testing

5. Start by covering the patient's left eye.
   Ensures consistency of testing

6. Record the last line read with no errors.

7. Repeat the procedure to test the left eye.

Procedure Notes:

Document on the Patient's Chart:

- Date and time
- Patient complaints or concerns
- Observations of patient during assessment, including with or without visual aids
- Jaegar results
- Your signature

EXAMPLE

7/23/2004	CC: c/o gradual onset of blurred near vi-
11:25 AM	sion OU. Jaegar exam performed, last
	line read with no errors is #7 OD, #6 OS.
	—S. Flowe, RMA

8

You Need to Know:

- If corrective lenses are worn for testing, record this on the patient's record.

Is a patient having trouble hearing?

Procedure 8-12

Performing Audiometry

1. Assemble this equipment:
   - Audiometer
   - Disposable scope cover

2. Follow these Standard Precautions.

3. Greet and identify the patient.

4. Escort the patient to a quiet room free of distractions.
   Eliminates extraneous sounds

5. Explain the procedure.

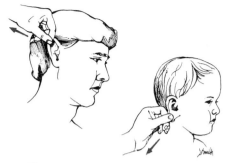

Figure 8-4. Position the ear as shown.

8

6. Cover the probe with the disposable scope cover.
   Prevents spread of microorganisms

7. Insert the probe into the patient's ear. Position the auricle and straighten the canal by gently pulling up and
   back on the pinna for adults, and by pulling gently
   down and back for small children (Figure 8-4). Visualize the tympanic membrane. Turn on the machine.
   Proper placement facilitates testing and helps ensure accurate results

8. Practice with the patient using the pretone.
   Ensures that the patient understands the instructions for testing

9. Select the testing level for the patient. Depress the
   "start" button. Observe the tone indicators and the patient's response.

10. Screen the opposite ear.
    Allows for bilateral testing

11. If the patient fails to respond at any frequency, repeat
    steps 7 to 10 to retest.
    Allows for assessment of the patient's failure to respond

12. Thank the patient for cooperating.

13. Remove and dispose of the probe cover. Wash your
    hands. Care for the equipment and return the instru-
    ment to its charging base.

Procedure Notes:

Document on the Patient's Chart:

- Date and time
- Patient complaints or concerns
- Physical findings
- Performance of procedure
- Testing results
- Patient education and instructions
- Your signature

EXAMPLE

4/14/2004	Audiometry performed as ordered for
10:15 AM	c/o diff. hearing. Pt. responded to mid-
	and low-level tones—failed to respond
	to upper-level tones. Test repeated
	with the same results obtained. Dr.
	Day notified of results.
	—V. Wang, RMA

You Need to Know:

- Visualizing the tympanic membrane before beginning the procedure ensures that the canal is not obstructed by cerumen or other objects.
- Adjust the probe securely in the patient's ear canal. An improperly secured probe does not provide a diagnostic test result.

Instruct the Patient or Caregiver Regarding:

- Placing objects in the ear for purposes of cleaning the canal; doing so may make the obstruction worse and may damage the tympanic membrane
- Safety precautions for young children who are likely to place small objects in the ear
- Protection against loud noises that can damage sensitive hearing receptors
- Importance of ear checks when signs of infection are present (e.g., tugging at the ears)

9

Vital Sign Assessment

Pulse

The most convenient site for assessing cardiac rhythm is also the most acceptable to patients.

Procedure 9-1

Measuring the Radial Pulse

1. Assemble this equipment:
   - Watch with sweep second hand

2. Follow these Standard Precautions.

3. Greet and identify the patient. Explain the procedure.

4. Place the patient in a seated or supine position with the arm relaxed and supported.
   Prevents altering pulse by ensuring appropriate position

5. With the index, middle, and ring fingers of the dominant hand, use the fingertips to press firmly enough to feel the pulse, but gently enough not to obliterate it.
   Increases probability of finding pulse with sensitive fingertips

6. If the pulse is regular, count it for 30 seconds and multiply by two. If this is a baseline pulse or if it is irregular, count for a full 60 seconds. Check at other sites if you are unsure of the assessment.
   Ensures accuracy

Document on the Patient's Chart:

- Date and time
- Patient complaints or concerns
- Heart rate at assessment site, rhythm, and volume
- Other observations appropriate to assessment of the cardiovascular system, such as skin color and skin temperature
- Other vital signs as needed or required by office protocol
- Your signature

EXAMPLE

09/24/2004	CC: c/o "racing heart beats" at
11:25 AM	times. Wt. 158# T 99 (o) P 96 reg
	R 16 BP 114/82 (L). Color pink, skin
	cool and dry.
	—C. Jones, CMA

Procedure Notes:

You Need to Know:

- Avoid using the thumb; it has a slight pulse of its own and may be confused with the patient's pulse. The thumb may be used on the opposite side of the patient's hand to steady the patient's hand and yours.
- If the radial pulse cannot be palpated, move to the apical pulse for an accurate measurement.
- Normal pulse ranges:

Birth to 1 year	110 to 170
1 to 10 years	90 to 110
10 to 16 years	80 to 95
16 years to midlife	70 to 80
Elderly adult	55 to 70

Should you assess this patient's pulse at the heart's apex?

Procedure 9-2

Measuring the Apical Pulse

1. Assemble this equipment:
   - Stethoscope
   - Watch with sweep second hand

2. Follow these Standard Precautions.

3. Greet and identify the patient. Explain the procedure.

9

4. Place the patient in a comfortable sitting or supine position. Remove the upper clothing or open sufficiently to allow access to the chest wall. Drape patient for privacy with a gown or sheet.

5. Locate the apex of the heart by palpating to the fifth intercostal space, between the fifth and sixth ribs. Move laterally to the left along the intercostal space to the nipple line or the midclavicular line (Figure 9-1).
   Locates cardiac apex, where sound is most likely to be heard

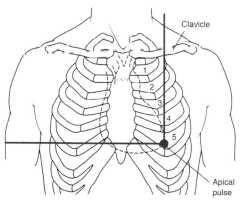

Figure 9-1. Finding the apical pulse site.

6. Clean the stethoscope diaphragm with alcohol and warm it in the palm of your hand.
   Prevents spread of microorganisms; avoids patient discomfort that may cause a rapid heart rate

7. Insert the earpieces into your ear canals with the openings pointing slightly forward.
   Facilitates sound transmission

8. Use a Doppler unit to amplify the heart sounds if they are difficult to discern, or to broadcast the sound.
   Amplifies sounds too faint to assess by palpation; broadcasting sound allows more than one worker to assess pulse

9. Listen for the S1 and S2 sinus sounds that sound like "lubb, dubb." Together, they count as one beat. "Lubb" sound indicates atrioventricular valve closure; "dubb" sound indicates semilunar valve closure.

10. Count beats for a full 60 seconds.
    Ensures accuracy in the presence of cardiovascular pathology

Procedure Notes:

9

You Need to Know:

- If the pulse must be measured at the apex, it may indicate that cardiovascular complications are present; therefore, the pulse should be measured for a full 60 seconds for an accurate reading.
- If cardiovascular disease is present, it may be necessary to compare the radial pulse with the apical pulse to evaluate the pulse deficit. This is the difference between the sounds heard at the apex and the pulse felt at the radius. If there is a difference, the apex is always the higher number. Generally, two people take the different pulses simultaneously, one at the apex, the other at the radius. With the watch at a point that both may see the sweep second hand, the apical recorder calls "start," usually as the hand reaches 12, 3, 6, or 9 to make it easier to keep track. The assistant who called "start" calls "stop" at the appropriate time, and the numbers are compared and recorded. If two workers are not available, one worker may perform the procedure by first counting one pulse for 60 seconds, then counting the other. Pulses measured in this manner are recorded as "apical/radial" or "A/R."
- Some offices may require that an apical pulse be assessed for all patients. All infants are assessed by the apical method.

Document on the Patient's Chart:

- Date and time
- Patient complaints or concerns
- Heart rate, rhythm, and volume
- Any observations appropriate for assessment of the cardiovascular system, such as skin color or skin temperature
- Other vital signs as needed or required by office protocol
- Patient education and instructions
- Your signature

EXAMPLE

11/06/2004	CC: BP recheck T 98.8 (o). Apical
2:15 PM	pulse 64 irreg, R 20 BP 104/62 (L).
	—K. Kriss, RMA

9

If the pulse cannot be palpated, the Doppler unit helps.

Procedure 9-3

Assessing the Pulse Using a Doppler Unit

1. Assemble this equipment:
   - Doppler unit
   - Coupling agent
   - Watch with sweep-second hand

2. Follow these Standard Precautions.

3. Use a generous amount of coupling agent or transmission gel on the probe to make an airtight seal.
   Promotes ultrasound transmission

Document on the Patient's Chart:

- Date and time
- Patient complaints or concerns
- Heart rate, rhythm, volume, location of assessment, use of Doppler unit
- Other observations appropriate to the cardiovascular system, such as skin color and skin temperature
- Other vitals as needed or required by office protocol
- Your signature

EXAMPLE

10/9/2004	CC: Postop check (R) knee replace-
12:20 PM	ment x10 days ago. No c/o pain,
	toes pink and warm with good
	movement, (R) pedal pulse per
	Doppler 88, reg.
	—R. Myers, RMA

4. With the machine on, hold the probe at a 45° angle with light pressure to ensure contact but to avoid obliterating the pulse (Figure 9-2). Arteries usually sound loud with a pumping sound; veins have a lighter, whooshing sound.

5. If the vein sound interferes with the measurement, reposition the probe until the artery sound is dominant.
   Facilitates assessment

6. Assess the rate, rhythm, and volume, and record the measurement.

7. Clean the patient's skin and the machine probe with warm water to remove the coupling gel.
   Ensures patient comfort

Procedure Notes:

Assessing the Pulse Using a Doppler Unit

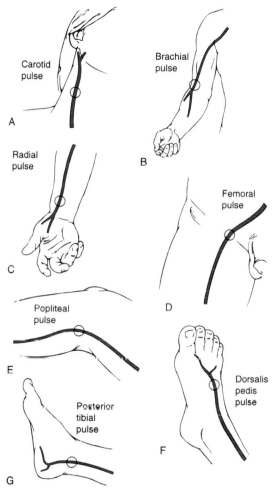

Figure 9-2. Sites for palpation of peripheral pulses.

You Need to Know:

- If the pulse must be measured using the Doppler unit, it may indicate that cardiovascular complications are present; therefore, the pulse should be measured for a full 60 seconds for an accurate reading.

Respirations
Assessment of respiratory function begins with this simple measure.

Procedure 9-4

Counting Respirations

1. Assemble this equipment:
   • Watch with sweep second hand

2. With patient already in position and sweep second hand in view after pulse procedure, count a complete rise and fall of the chest as one respiration.
   Ensures accurate measurement

3. If the pattern is regular, count respirations for 30 seconds and multiply by two, or count for 15 seconds and multiply by four. If the pattern is irregular, count respirations for a full 60 seconds.
   Ensures accuracy if rate is irregular

Procedure Notes:

You Need to Know:

• Normal ranges for respirations:

Infant	20+
Child	18 to 20
Adult	14 to 20

• Some patients breathe at rest using the abdominal muscles more than the chest muscles. Observe carefully for the easiest area to assess for the most accurate reading.

• Be aware of abnormal respiratory patterns, as described in Table 9-1.

Document on the Patient's Chart:

- Date and time
- Patient complaints or concerns
- Respiratory rate, rhythm, volume, and breath sounds
- Other observations appropriate to assessment of respiratory function, such as position assumed, effort required, and so on
- Other vital signs as needed or required by office protocol
- Patient education and instructions
- Your signature

EXAMPLE

7/9/2004	CC: c/o SOB with pain on inspira-
11:20 AM	tion, dyspnea when supine T: 99.4
	(o), P: 112 reg, R: 26, BP: 136/92
	(L). Color pale and pink, skin warm
	and dry. Dr. Morton notified.
	—J. Thomas, CMA

9

Table 9-1

Abnormal Respiratory Patterns

Pattern	Description
Apnea	No respirations
Bradypnea	Slow respirations
Cheyne-Stokes	Rhythmic cycles of dyspnea or hyperpnea subsiding gradually into periods of apnea
Dyspnea	Difficult or labored respirations
Hypopnea	Shallow respirations
Hyperpnea	Deep respirations
Kussmaul	Fast and deep respirations
Orthopnea	Inability to breathe in other than a sitting or standing position
Tachypnea	Fast respirations

Temperature

The axillary method of temperature measurement may be used if the oral method is contraindicated.

Procedure 9-5

Measuring Axillary Temperature Using a Glass Mercury Thermometer

1. Assemble this equipment:
   - Glass mercury thermometer, either oral or rectal, according to facility's policy
   - Tissues or cotton balls
   - Sheath, if used

2. Follow these Standard Precautions.

3. Check the thermometer for chips or cracks.
   Ensures patient safety

4. Greet and identify the patient. Explain the procedure.
   Prevents errors in treatment; eases anxiety and ensures compliance

5. Rinse and dry the thermometer if it has been stored in solution. Wipe from stem to bulb.

6. Read the thermometer by holding it by the stem horizontal to your face and turning it slowly to see the mercury column.
   Makes it easier to visualize column

7. If the thermometer registers above 94°F, grasp the thermometer by the stem with the thumb and forefinger and snap the wrist quickly several times to shake the mercury down to about 94°F. Avoid hitting the thermometer against anything.
   Returns mercury to lowest mark to reduce errors; prevents breakage

8. If using a clear plastic sheath, cover the thermometer now. Follow package directions for application.
   Reduces number of microorganisms on thermometer

9. Expose the axillary area. Do not expose more of the patient's chest or upper body than is necessary to ensure the proper placement of the thermometer.
Maintains privacy

10. Dry the axilla with patting motions, because friction increases surface temperature.
Prevents axillary moisture that may cause thermometer to slip

11. Place the bulb of the thermometer well into the axilla. Close the arm down over the axilla and cross the forearm over the chest. Drape the clothes or gown over the patient for privacy.
Offers the best exposure to the mercury column and maintains a closed environment; prevents exposing patient unnecessarily

12. Leave the thermometer in place for 10 minutes. Stay with the patient.
Assures proper time to register; ensures compliance

13. Remove the thermometer after the prescribed time. Remove the sheath or clean from stem to bulb, cleaning from cleanest area to less clean area. Note the reading.
Prevents surface dirt or perspiration from obscuring mercury column

14. Thank the patient and provide appropriate instructions.

15. Disinfect the thermometer according to the facility's policy. Wash your hands.

Procedure Notes:

You Need to Know:

- This is an excellent method for assessing a child's temperature but is time consuming and requires that the child remain still. Have the parent hold the child with the arm holding the thermometer against the parent's body to keep the thermometer in place. The parent may read to the child during this time or may give the child a bottle, if appropriate.
- In offices that do not use the tympanic temperature measurement, this is the preferred method for assessing the temperature of patients under the age of 2 months to avoid damage to the rectal canal.

Table 9-2		
Temperature Comparisons		
	Fahrenheit	**Centigrade**
Oral	98.6°	37.0°
Rectal	99.6° (R)	37.6°
Axillary	97.6° (A)	36.4°
Tympanic	98.6° (T)	37.0°

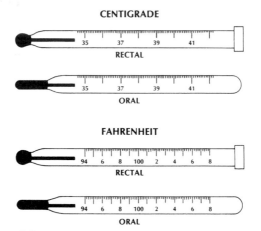

Figure 9-3. The two glass thermometers on the top use the centigrade scale to measure temperature; the two on the bottom use the Fahrenheit scale. Note the blunt bulbs on the rectal thermometers and the long thin bulbs on the oral thermometers.

- Be aware of normal body temperatures, as measured via various routes (Table 9-2).
- If the physician prefers centigrade to Fahrenheit, or vice versa, the thermometer provided should be in the preferred measurement (Figure 9-3).
- If it is necessary to convert from centigrade to Fahrenheit or vice versa, use this rule:
  —To convert centigrade to Fahrenheit, multiply the number of degrees centigrade by $\frac{9}{5}$ and add 32 to the result.
  —To convert Fahrenheit to centigrade, subtract 32 from the number of degrees and multiply the difference by 5/9.

Document on the Patient's Chart:

- Date and time
- Patient complaints or concerns
- Temperature, indicate axillary with (A)
- Other vital signs as needed or required by office protocol
- Patient education and instructions
- Your signature

EXAMPLE

07/09/2004	CC: Mother states 8-month-old
8:35 AM	congested x3 days, tugging at AS
	x1 day, denies fever T. 100.6 (Ax)
	P 124 R 32.
	—J. Bunch, CMA

9

Instruct the Patient or Caregiver to:

- Dry the axilla and hold the arm close to the body
- Create and maintain a strong seal at the axilla
- Hold and feed or rock a child during the procedure

Is the patient complaining of fever symptoms? Does routine examination protocol require temperature assessment?

Procedure 9-6

Measuring Oral Temperature Using a Glass Mercury Thermometer

1. Assemble this equipment:
   - Glass mercury thermometer designed for oral use
   - Tissues or cotton balls
   - Disposable plastic sheath, if used

2. Follow these Standard Precautions.

3. Check the thermometer for chips or cracks.
Ensures safety

4. Greet and identify the patient. Explain the procedure. Check for recent eating, drinking, gum chewing, or smoking.
Reduces risk of altered reading

5. Rinse and dry the thermometer if it has been stored in solution. Wipe from stem to bulb.
Prevents irritating oral mucosa

6. Read the thermometer by holding it by the stem horizontal to your face and turning it slowly to see the mercury column.
Makes it easier to visualize column; prevents touching bulb, which will be inserted in patient's mouth

7. If the thermometer registers above 94°F, grasp the thermometer by the stem with the thumb and forefinger and snap the wrist quickly several times to shake the mercury down to about 94°F. Avoid hitting the thermometer against anything.
Returns mercury to lowest mark to reduce errors; prevents breakage

8. If using a clear plastic sheath, cover the thermometer now. Follow package directions for application.
Reduces number of microorganisms on thermometer

9. Put on gloves.
Prevents exposure to body fluid

10. Place the thermometer under the tongue to either side of the frenulum.
Ensures most accurate reading due to high vascularity in the area

11. Tell the patient to keep his mouth closed, but caution against biting down on the glass column.
Prevents cooler air from entering the mouth, reduces risk of breaking thermometer

12. Leave the thermometer in place for 3 to 5 minutes.
Allows mercury column to register body temperature

13. Remove the thermometer after the prescribed time. Remove and discard the sheath, if used, in the proper container, or wipe the thermometer with a clean tissue or cotton ball from stem to bulb. Wipe from clean to less clean area.

Prevents obscuring column by mucus or sheath

14. Hold the thermometer as before and note the reading.

15. Thank the patient and provide appropriate instructions.

16. Disinfect the thermometer according to the facility's policy. Remove gloves. Wash your hands.

Procedure Notes:

9

WARNING!

Do not attempt to take an oral temperature on patients who are post-operative for oral surgery, have seizure disorders, are receiving oxygen, are mouth breathers or are congested, or for small children.

You Need to Know:

• The pulse and respirations may be taken during this time.
• Leave the thermometer in for 3 minutes if there is no evidence of fever and the patient is compliant. Leave in for 5 minutes if the patient is febrile or noncompliant.

Instruct the Patient or Caregiver Regarding:

• Current theories that suggest temperature elevations are a natural response to disease processes and that efforts to lower the temperature may be counterproductive
• The need to bring the temperature to about 101°F to ensure the patient's comfort; however, the patient should not expect the temperature to return to normal until the illness has run its course
• Comfort measures, which include resting, eating a light diet, consuming clear liquids if nausea and vomiting are present, and avoiding chilling
• The use of a nonaspirin antipyretic as needed for comfort, because aspirin has been implicated in Reye syndrome in certain populations

Document on the Patient's Chart:

- Date and time
- Patient complaints or concerns
- Temperature, indicate by mouth (O), if necessary
- Other vital signs as needed or required by office protocol
- Patient education and instructions
- Your signature

1/14/2004	CC: c/o "flu symptoms" x3 days in-
4:10 PM	cluding "slight fever, aching joints".
	T 101.6 (O) P 94 reg R 22 BP
	104/62 (R).
	—R. Torres, RMA

What should you do if other methods of temperature assessment are inappropriate for a patient?

Procedure 9-7

Measuring Rectal Temperature Using a Glass Mercury Thermometer

1. Assemble this equipment:
   - Glass mercury thermometer designed for rectal use
   - Surgical lubricant
   - Tissues
   - Disposable plastic sheath, if used

2. Follow these Standard Precautions.

3. Check the thermometer for chips or cracks.
   Ensures patient safety

4. Greet and identify the patient. Explain the procedure.

5. Rinse and dry the thermometer if it has been stored in solution. Wipe from stem to bulb.

6. Read the thermometer by holding it by the stem horizontal to your face and turning it slowly to see the mercury column.
   Makes it easier to visualize column

7. If the thermometer registers above 94°F, grasp the thermometer by the stem with the thumb and forefinger and snap the wrist quickly several times to shake the mercury down to about 94°F. Avoid hitting the thermometer against anything.
   Returns mercury to lowest mark to reduce errors; prevents breakage

9

8. If using a clear plastic sheath, cover the thermometer now. Follow package directions for application.
   Reduces number of microorganisms on thermometer

9. Spread lubricant onto a tissue, then from the tissue to the thermometer. Put on gloves.
   Prevents spread of pathogens to tube of lubricant; lubricants for rectal insertion prevent patient discomfort

10. Ensure privacy. Place the patient in a side-lying position to expose anus. Make sure patient is facing toward the examination room door. Drape appropriately.
    Prevents embarrassment for the patient if door is opened inadvertently; diminishes chance of exposure

11. Expose only the buttock area. With the nondominant hand, lift the topmost buttock. Visualize the anus.
    Prevents exposing patient unnecessarily; ensures clear view of anus

12. Touch the thermometer to the anus lightly. The anus usually tightens reflexively against the intrusion. When the anus relaxes, insert the thermometer gently past the sphincter. Have the patient breathe deeply with the mouth opened.
    Reduces risk of perforating rectal canal; breathing through the mouth relaxes the patient

13. Insert the thermometer about $1\frac{1}{2}$ inches for an adult, 1 inch for a child, and $\frac{1}{2}$ inch for an infant over the age of 2 months.

Reduces risk of perforating rectal canal

14. Release the upper buttock and drape the sheet back over the patent. Hold the thermometer in place for 3 minutes.

Maintains patient privacy; keeps thermometer from falling out

15. At the end of 3 minutes, remove the thermometer. Offer the patient a tissue for cleaning or assist as needed. Wipe the thermometer from stem to bulb or remove the sheath if used by turning it inside out as it is pulled from the thermometer. Discard the sheath in the appropriate container.

Avoids patient discomfort; prevents obscuring mercury column by lubricant or sheath; reduces transmission of pathogens

16. Note the reading. Remove and dispose of gloves. Wash your hands.

17. Thank the patient and provide appropriate instructions.

18. Disinfect thermometer according to the facility's policy. Wash your hands.

Procedure Notes:

WARNING!

· *Rectal temperatures should not be attempted for postoperative rectal surgery patients, for patients with cardiac or seizure disorders, or for children under the age of 2 months.*

· *Infants under the age of 2 months should have temperatures taken by the axillary or tympanic method to avoid damage to the rectal canal.*

You Need to Know:

• Infants over the age of 2 months and very small children may be held in the lap or over the knees for this procedure, or they may

Document on the Patient's Chart:

- Date and time
- Patient complaints or concerns
- Temperature; indicate rectal with (R)
- Other vital signs as needed or required by office protocol
- Patient education and instructions
- Your signature

EXAMPLE

6/24/2004	CC: 2½-year-old with history of ex-
9:45 AM	posure to chickenpox, rash over
	trunk x2 days per mother.
	T 101.4 (R) P 114 R 30.
	—C. Smith, CMA

9

remain on the examining table with the parent close by. Hold the thermometer and the buttocks with the dominant hand while securing the child with nondominant hand. If the child moves with the thermometer in place, the thermometer and the hand will move together with the buttocks and avoid perforating the rectal canal.

Instruct the Patient or Caregiver to:

- Practice good hygiene to avoid the spread of pathogens
- Follow these guidelines for insertion depths:

Adult	1½ inches
Child	1 inch
Infant over 2 months	½ inch

- Use a water-soluble lubricant rather than petrolatum to avoid damage to the rectal canal
- Apply the lubricant to a tissue rather than to the thermometer to avoid the spread of pathogens
- Avoid trauma to the rectal canal by never forcing the thermometer insertion

This method of temperature assessment is rapidly gaining favor with both health care professionals and patients.

Procedure 9-8

Measuring Temperature Using an Electronic Thermometer

1. Assemble this equipment:
   - Battery-powered unit with probes and covers
   - Gloves
   - Lubricant for rectal temperature

2. Follow these Standard Precautions.

(as needed)

3. Greet and identify the patient. Explain the procedure.

4. Choose the method most appropriate for the particular patient (e.g., oral, rectal, axillary) and cover the probe to be used. Almost all units have one probe for oral and one for rectal. Covers are carried with the unit in a specially fitted box attached to the back of the unit. Adhere to facility policy for the appropriate method for the patient.

5. Place the thermometer as described for measuring an oral temperature, rectal temperature, or axillary temperature. Glove if the measurement of choice is rectal.

6. If taking an oral temperature, help the patient hold the probe. If taking a rectal temperature, you must hold the probe.
   Assists patient in holding heavy probe

7. Note that the electronic unit emits a beep when the temperature shows no signs of rising beyond the point reached. This is usually within 20 to 60 seconds.

8. Remove the probe from the patient. Note the reading; most units retain the reading until the probe is reinserted into the unit.

Document on the Patient's Chart:

- Date and time
- Patient complaints or concerns
- Temperature; indicate axillary with (A), rectal with (R)
- Other vital signs as needed or required by office protocol
- Patient education and instructions
- Your signature

EXAMPLE

01/05/2004	CC: sore throat x2 days. Has used
1:15 PM	OTC throat lozenges and aspirin
	without relief. Skin warm and
	flushed. T 101.4 (O) P 96 reg R 24
	BP 122/74 (L).
	—R. Winston CMA

9

9. Discard the probe cover in a waste receptacle. Insert the probe into its holder in the unit. If this was a rectal temperature, help the patient to clean away any remaining lubricant.

10. Remove gloves. Wash your hands.

11. Return the unit to the charging base.
    Ensures unit is charged and ready for use

Procedure Notes:

You Need to Know:

- Electronic thermometers do not require the time limits set for glass thermometers. Most provide a reading in well under 60 seconds.

This quick and easy method of assessing body temperature is readily accepted by most patients.

Procedure 9-9

Measuring Temperature Using a Tympanic Thermometer

1. Assemble this equipment:
   - Tympanic thermometer
   - Disposable probe covers

2. Follow these Standard Precautions.

3. Greet and identify the patient. Explain the procedure.

4. Remove the tympanic thermometer from the base and put the disposable cover on the probe.

5. Insert the probe, sealing the opening of the ear canal. Press the button to take the temperature, which is displayed on the digital screen in about 2 seconds.

6. Remove the probe and note the reading. Discard the probe cover in a waste receptacle.
   Avoids exposure to the contaminated probe cover

7. Thank the patient and provide appropriate instructions.
   Encourages a positive attitude about office and physician

8. Return the unit to the base for recharge.

Procedure Notes:

You Need to Know:

- Electronic thermometers do not require the time limits set for glass thermometers. Most provide a reading in about 2 to 5 seconds.

Document on the Patient's Chart:
- Date and time
- Patient complaints or concerns
- Temperature; indicate tympanic with (T)
- Other vital signs as needed or required by office protocol
- Patient education and instructions
- Your signature

EXAMPLE

04/16/2004	CC: 8-month-old listless and fever-
1:20 PM	ish since last PM. Per mom, appetite
	poor x2 days. x3 loose stools since
	yesterday, no emesis. Skin flushed
	and moist. Wt. 20 3/4 # T: 101.3 (T),
	P: 124, R 30.
	—J. Clifton, RMA

9

Blood Pressure
Measuring the force of blood flow through the body is an important evaluation measure for cardiac function.

Procedure 9-10

Measuring Adult Blood Pressure

1. Assemble this equipment:
   - Sphygmomanometer
   - Stethoscope
   - Alcohol wipe
2. Follow these Standard Precautions.

3. Identify the patient and explain the procedure. Ask the patient about recent smoking, caffeine, exercise, or emotional upset.
Reduces factors that affect pressure levels

4. Position the patient. Have the patient's arm supported and slightly flexed with the palm upward. The upper arm should be level with the heart. The patient's legs should not be crossed, and the feet should be flat on the floor.
Makes palpating the brachial artery easier; ensures accurate pressure reading

5. Expose the area. Remove the garment if the sleeve is too tight to raise above the area.
Prevents tight clothing acting as a tourniquet or obscuring sound transmission

6. Center the deflated cuff over the brachial artery (Figure 9-4) on the medial aspect of the upper arm. To assess the center of the cuff, fold the bladder in half; place the midpoint just above the brachial artery. The lower edge of the cuff should be 1 to 2 inches above the antecubital area.
Positions cuff over artery for correct reading

7. Wrap the cuff smoothly. It should fit snugly against the arm without being too tight. Cuffs vary. Cuffs may fasten with Velcro, hooks, or long cloth tails.
Ensures even pressure for an accurate reading

8. If using a mercury manometer, keep it vertical and at eye level. An aneroid dial must register with the needle at zero before beginning.
Ensures accurate reading

9. Palpate the brachial pulse with the fingertips of the nondominant hand in the antecubital area.
Locates pulse for most accurate reading

10. With air pump in the dominant hand and valve between the thumb and forefinger, turn the screw clockwise right to tighten. Do not tighten it to the point that it is difficult to release.
Allows cuff to fill properly; prevents difficulty in opening valve at completion of procedure

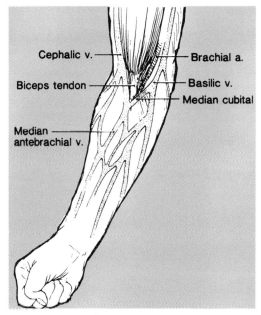

Figure 9-4. Finding the brachial artery.

11. With the fingers of the nondominant hand still at the pulse, inflate the cuff and note the point at which the brachial pulse is no longer felt. This number is slightly below the first Korotkoff sound heard on auscultation.
Gives reference point for accessing pressure and goal for reinflating cuff

12. Deflate the cuff by turning the knob counterclockwise (left to loosen). Wait at least 30 seconds before reinflating the cuff. The patient may raise or flex the arm and hand briefly to restore full circulation.
Allows circulation to return to normal

13. Clean the stethoscope chest piece with alcohol.
Prevents cross-contamination

14. Place the stethoscope earpieces in your ear canals with the openings pointing slightly forward.
Facilitates sound transmission to ear canals

15. Stand or sit about 3 feet from the manometer, with the gauge at eye level. The stethoscope tubing should hang freely and should not rub against anything.
Reduces errors in visualizing or determining reading

16. Place the bell or diaphragm against the brachial artery, but do not press hard. Hold with the nondominant hand.
Ensures correct placement and proper sound transmission

17. With the valve in the dominant hand, thumb and forefinger on the valve screw, turn the screw just tightly enough to inflate the cuff. Pump the valve to about 30 mmHg above the number felt on palpation.
Prevents difficulty in releasing the air from the pump; avoids patient discomfort from overinflated cuff

18. With the thumb and forefinger remaining on the screw, slowly release the air at about 2 to 4 mmHg per second.
Prevents missed beats or interfering with circulation

19. Listening carefully, note the point on the gauge at which the first clear tapping sound is heard. This is the first systolic sound, or Korotkoff I (Table 9-3).

20. Read at the top level of the meniscus (curved surface) of the mercury or at the number indicated by an arrow on the aneroid. Aneroid and mercury measurements are usually recorded as even numbers.
Ensures accurate measurement

21. Maintaining control of the valve screw, continue to deflate at about 2 to 4 mmHg per second and identify each of the Korotkoff sounds.

Table 9-3

Five Phases of Blood Pressure

Phase	Sounds
I	Faint tapping sounds heard as the cuff deflates (systolic)
II	Soft swishing sounds
III	Rhythmic, sharp, distinct tapping sounds
IV	Soft tapping sounds that become faint
V	No sounds (diastolic)

22. When the last sound is heard, note the reading and quickly deflate the cuff.
Identifies diastolic, or Korotkoff V, sound

23. Remove the cuff and press the air from the bladder.

24. If this is the first recording or the first patient visit, be aware that the physician may want a reading in the opposite arm also, or in a position other than sitting.
Ensures that all variables are assessed and recorded

25. Clean and store the equipment. Wash your hands.

Procedure Notes:

9

WARNING!

· *Never attempt to assess pressure in a patient's arm used for a dialysis shunt. Avoid limbs with edema, a heparin lock, or injuries of any sort. If possible, avoid using the affected arm after a mastectomy.*
· *Notify the physician immediately if the pressure reads above 140/90 or below 100/50. Check in both arms if the pressure is very high or low.*
· *Never immediately reinflate the cuff if you are unsure of the reading. Totally deflate the cuff and wait at least 1 minute before repeating the procedure. Have the patient raise her arm and flex the fingers of that hand to restore circulation and relieve vasocongestion if the pressure must be reassessed.*

You Need to Know:

- Many physicians require that all sounds be recorded rather than the traditional systolic/diastolic measurements.
- The palpatory method may be used if the Korotkoff sounds cannot be heard. Using the properly placed cuff, pump 30 mmHg above the last felt pulse. Watching the mercury column or the aneroid needle as it drops, record the number at which the systolic pulse is felt at the radius. The diastolic pressure cannot be assessed in this manner.
- Have patient sitting unless the physician specifies a standing or lying pressure assessment. Always record the position if it is other than sitting.

BOX 9-1

Causes of Errors in Blood Pressure Readings

- Wrapping the cuff improperly
- Failing to keep the patient's arm at heart level
- Failing to support the patient's arm on a stable surface
- Recording auscultatory gap for diastolic pressure
- Failing to maintain the gauge at eye level
- Pulling the patient's sleeve up tightly above the cuff
- Listening through clothing
- Allowing the cuff to deflate too rapidly or too slowly
- Failing to wait 1 to 2 minutes before rechecking

9

- If the upper arm is higher than heart level, the pressure readings will be inaccurate. If the legs are crossed, the pressure may be higher than normal.
- If the cuff is too low on the arm, it may interfere with the stethoscope placement and increase the environmental noises, obscuring the pressure sounds.
- If the meniscus of the mercury is read at other than eye level, the reading may be falsely high or low.
- If the aneroid needle does not register zero, it should not be used until professionally calibrated.
- The bell magnifies low-pitched sounds better than the diaphragm. The diaphragm covers more area, which may assist with finding the pulse if the brachial pulse has been hard to palpate. If not pressed firmly enough, the sounds may not be heard; if pressed too firmly, the pulse may be obliterated.
- Inflating more than 30 mmHg over the palpated pressure point is uncomfortable for the patient and is unnecessary; inflating less than 30 mmHg may cause the highest systolic reading to be missed.
- Be aware that a number of factors may result in incorrect blood pressure readings (Box 9-1). Instruct the Patient or Caregiver to:
- Discuss concerns about pressure with his or her physician
- Follow prudent living guidelines as outlined by a dietitian or nutritionist

Document on the Patient's Chart:

- Date and time
- Patient complaints or concerns
- Pressure reading and observations such as patient position, if other than sitting, and arm used. Record the result, with the systolic over the diastolic.
- Record other vital signs as needed or required by office protocol
- Actions taken, if needed
- Patient education and instructions
- Your signature

EXAMPLE

01/12/2004	CC: c/o headache x3 days, worse to-
2:00 PM	day. Has taken aspirin without relief.
	BP 180/120 (L). Dr. Rodriquez
	notified.
	—S. Gomez, CMA

- Follow these guidelines for home assessment of pressure:
  - —Support the arm, slightly flexed, palm up
  - —If sitting, have both feet on the floor
  - —Place the cuff at heart level
  - —Expose the arm, but do not push the sleeve up tightly
  - —Wrap the cuff smoothly
  - —Unless otherwise prescribed, always use the same arm

10

Emergency Procedures

What should you do when a patient has a seizure?

Procedure 10-1

Caring for a Patient During a Seizure

1. If the patient is sitting or standing, help the patient to the floor and remove nearby objects, chairs, tables, and so forth.
   Prevents injury from falling or from striking nearby objects

2. Protect the patient's head and limbs, but do not restrain the patient.
   Prevents injury to patient from thrashing about

3. Provide privacy for the patient.
   Prevents additional embarrassment

4. Alert the physician immediately, because decisions must be made regarding hospitalization, medications, and so on.

5. Place the patient in the recovery position (side-lying) when the seizure is over (Figure 10-1).
   Prevents aspiration of excessive saliva or vomitus

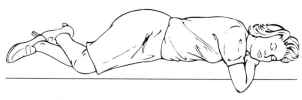

Figure 10-1. Patient in recovery position.

Document on the Patient's Chart:

- Date and time
- Onset characteristics or precipitating factors
- Duration of seizure
- Characteristics of seizure
- Vital signs
- Postseizure procedures
- Your signature

10

11/28/2004	Pt. notified receptionist of an aura
10:25 AM	of flashing lights that is often
	seen "before a seizure". Clinical
	staff notified immediately & pt.
	escorted to exam room, assisted
	to supine position on the floor. Dr.
	Miranda notified. Seizure activity
	started at 10:30 AM with general-
	ized hand, arm, and leg tremors—
	lasted 3 min. Postseizure VS P 96
	reg R 24 BP 136/88 (R) emer-
	gency medical services (EMS) no-
	tified, pt. transferred to Metropoli-
	tan Hospital.
	—M. Perkins, CMA

Performing Cardiopulmonary Resuscitation

Procedure Notes:

> ### WARNING!
>
> *Do not put anything in the patient's mouth. He will not "swallow" his tongue. Trying to force objects through a tightly clenched jaw may damage teeth or tongue or may cause aspiration of the object.*

You Need to Know:

- A seizure may be frightening to you and to other patients. Maintain professionalism at all times. If the seizure occurs in the reception area, have someone escort the waiting patients to another area or provide a screen for the seizing patient.

Instruct the Patient or Caregiver to:

- Remember the aura warning sign and to report it to the physician
- Time the seizure, if possible, and describe its onset and character
- Provide for the patient's safety as described above
- Take or administer seizure medication as instructed even in the absence of seizure activity

How should you handle a cardiac arrest?

Procedure 10-2

Performing Cardiopulmonary Resuscitation (CPR) (One Rescuer)

1. If time allows, assemble this equipment:
   - Barrier respiratory devices
   - If time permits in an out-of-office emergency, secure barrier devices such as gloves and a respiratory device for your protection. These are available in the office situation on the crash cart or tray.

2. Establish patient unresponsiveness by shaking the patient and shouting "Are you OK?"
   Prevents performing rescue measures unnecessarily

3. Activate the EMS system if there is no response.
   Increases chances of patient's survival

4. Position the patient in supine position with head level with body, and kneel by patient's shoulders.
Assists with restoring blood flow to brain; makes compressions more effective

5. Open the airway with the head-tilt, chin-lift maneuver (Figure 10-2).
Determines respiratory status

6. Determine breathlessness by looking, listening, and feeling for breaths.
Avoids giving respirations to breathing patients

7. If the patient is breathing and her condition allows, place her in the recovery position (refer to Figure 10-1) until consciousness returns or help arrives.
Facilitates respirations and avoids aspiration of vomitus

8. If the patient is not breathing, maintain head-tilt, chin-lift and give two slow breaths just until the chest rises.
Provides oxygen to patient without overfilling the lung fields and causing gastric distension or vomiting

9. Check the carotid pulse. If no pulse is present, locate the xiphocostal notch, and place the long axis of the nondominant palm on the sternum two fingers above the notch (Figure 10-3). Lace the fingers, with the dominant hand pressing against the back of the non-dominant hand at the proper position.

10

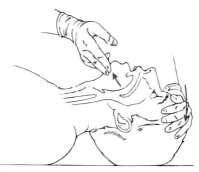

Figure 10-2. The head-tilt/chin-lift technique. The head is tilted backward with one hand (down arrow), while the fingers of the other hand lift the chin forward (up arrow).

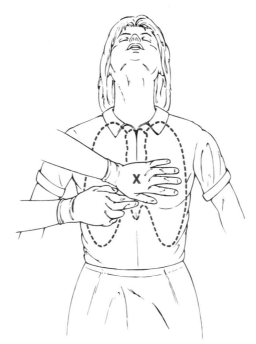

Figure 10-3. Place the long axis of the nondominant palm on the sternum two fingers above the xiphocostal notch.

10. With the upper body perpendicular to the patient's chest, rock from the hips with the force of the upper body and stiffened arms compressing the sternum 1½ to 2 inches (Figure 10-4). Keep the hands at position during the upstroke, but allow the chest to expand completely before the next compression. Give cycles of 15 chest compressions and 2 breaths at a rate of 80 to 100 per minute (four cycles per minute).

11. After giving four cycles of 15 chest compressions and 2 breaths in about 1 minute, check the patient's carotid pulse. If no pulse is present, continue the 15:2 cycle beginning with chest compressions. Continue until help arrives or until a pulse is present at the pulse

check. If the pulse returns but respirations do not, continue giving breaths at 14 to 16 per minute until help arrives. Transport patient to an emergency facility.

Procedure Notes:

WARNING!

· *The physician or trained medical assistant may use an automatic external defibrillator (AED) machine to convert the patient's heart rhythm. Stand clear of the patient when the rescuer activates the machine and follow all instructions.*

· *In the clinical situation, respiratory devices are available to protect you from the patient's oral secretions. In an out-of-office situation, these protective devices may not be at hand.*

10

You Need to Know:

· For detailed coverage of CPR and assessment of proficiency, apply for certification through your local American Heart Association or Red Cross chapter.

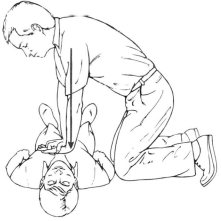

Figure 10-4. Compress the sternum.

Document on the Patient's Chart:

- Date and time
- Description of incident
- Time CPR was initiated
- Time that EMS arrived
- Hospital destination
- Notification of physician
- Your signature

EXAMPLE

9/3/2004	During ECG, pt. c/o chest pain VS P
9:45 AM	144 reg R 32 BP 136/98. Dr. Baker
	notified. Cardiac arrest at 9:55 AM.
	CPR started by Dr. Baker with as-
	sistance from D. Mendez, CMA. AED
	applied, shock delivered at 10:00 AM,
	sinus rhythm restored. EMS arrived
	at 10:12. Pt. transported to Metro-
	politan Hospital at 10:25 AM.
	—C. Brown, CMA

- Maintain current certification through a qualified instructor. Skills infrequently used are quickly forgotten; frequent recertification (at least annually) reinforces sequencing and proper technique.
- Nonclinical personnel should be instructed to call the EMS, and those who have been trained in CPR begin the procedure.
- Post current flow charts and algorithms in prominent areas.
- Know how to use the available barrier devices.
- Know the location of your emergency cart or tray, and be familiar with its contents and their use.
- Reassure and comfort family members and patients who might be aware of the emergency.

How should you help a patient who is choking?

Procedure 10-3

Managing an Adult Patient With a Foreign Body Airway Obstruction

1. If time allows, assemble this equipment:
   - Barrier respiratory devices
   - If time permits in an out-of-office emergency, secure barrier devices such as gloves and a respiratory device for your protection. These are available in the office situation on the crash cart or tray.

2. Ask the patient, "Are you choking?" If the patient is able to speak or cough, the obstruction is not complete. Observe for increased distress and assist the patient as needed, but do not perform thrusts.
   Prevents injury to patient who is not in need of assistance

10

3. If the patient is unable to speak or cough and is displaying the universal sign for distress, stand behind the patient; wrap your arms around his waist; make a fist with the nondominant hand, thumb side against the abdomen at midline between navel and xiphoid. Grasp fist with dominant hand and give quick upward abdominal thrusts (Figure 10-5). Completely relax arms between each thrust, and make each thrust forceful enough to relieve obstruction.
   Forces air upward from lungs into airway with enough pressure to expel foreign body

4. Repeat thrusts until effective or until the victim becomes unconscious.
   Provides assistance necessary to expel object

5. If the victim is unconscious, or becomes unconscious, activate the EMS system.
   Summons emergency personnel to provide assistance

6. Put on gloves now if available. Perform a tongue-jaw lift followed by a finger sweep to remove the object. (The object may become visible with loss of consciousness and may be removed.)

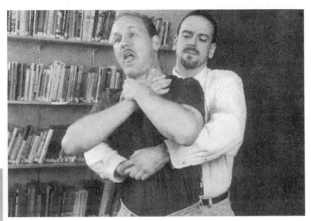

10

Figure 10-5. Give abdominal thrusts.

7. Open the airway and try to ventilate (Figure 10-6). If the airway is still obstructed, reposition the patient's head and try to ventilate again. Use a barrier respiratory device if available.
Ensures that airway obstruction is not caused by improper head position

8. If the air is still not expanding the lungs, straddle the patient's hips. Place the long axis of your nondominant palm between the patient's navel and xiphoid process; lace your fingers with the dominant hand against the back of the properly positioned nondominant hand. Give up to five upward abdominal thrusts.
May expel object

9. Repeat steps 6 through 8 until effective.

Procedure Notes:

Managing a Foreign Body Airway Obstruction

You Need to Know:

- For detailed coverage of foreign body airway obstruction (FBAO) management and assessment of proficiency, apply for Health Care Provider certification through your local American Heart Association or Red Cross.
- If gloves are available in an emergency that you encounter outside of the office, put them on before doing a finger sweep to avoid exposure to oral secretions. Use your judgment in an out-of-office situation if barrier respiratory devices are not available.

- If the patient is significantly taller than you are, it may be necessary to have the patient sit or to raise yourself to a higher position by stepping up on a stool or other object. It is very difficult to achieve the proper effective upward angle for abdominal thrusts from a height lower than the patient's height.
- Obese or pregnant patients require chest thrusts rather than abdominal thrusts.
- Children over the age of 8 years are considered to be adults for the purposes of FBAO management.

Instruct the Patient to:

- Chew food thoroughly and use caution while swallowing; this is particularly important for those with loose-fitting dentures or dysphagia, and for those who drink alcoholic beverages

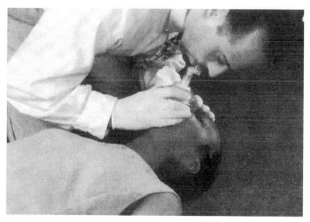

Figure 10-6. Try to ventilate the patient.

Document on the Patient's Chart:

- Date and time
- Description of the incident that led to FBAO
- Number of thrusts required to dislodge the object
- Object's nature and approximate size
- Any signs or symptoms of respiratory distress
- Notification of the physician
- Patient education, if appropriate
- Action taken at completion of emergency
- Your signature

EXAMPLE

8/5/2004	Pt. choked on throat lozenge while
11:05 AM	in reception area. Coughing noted
	at first, complete obstruction with
	no air movement after x2-3 at-
	tempts at removal during cough-
	ing. x6 abd. thrusts given, lozenge
	ejected after pt. vomited.
	Dr. Kramer notified. VS P 112, reg R
	36 BP 118/76 (L).
	—L. Ravell, CMA

Table 10-1

Is It Angina or Myocardial Infarction?

The pain felt with angina and myocardial infarction is brought about by myocardial anoxia, which is caused by an increased need for oxygen to the heart muscle because of exertion, stress, or temperature extremes of heat or cold. Typically, angina may be relieved by rest or nitroglycerin. However, pain from a myocardial infarction is not relieved by these measures. Here is a brief comparison of these two disorders.

	Angina	Myocardial Infarction
Description	Moderate pressure felt deeply in the chest; a squeezing, suffocating feeling.	Severe deep pressure not relieved by reducing stressors; a crushing pressure.
Onset	Pain may occur gradually or suddenly and subsides quickly, usually in less than 30 minutes. It can be relieved by reducing the stressors, by rest, and by nitroglycerin protocol.	Pain occurs suddenly and remains even after stressors are reduced or relieved. Pain is not relieved by nitroglycerin, which may be given up to three times, one dose every 5 minutes for a total of three doses in 15 minutes.
Location	Mid-anterior chest, usually diffuse; radiates to the back, neck, arms, jaw, and epigastric area.	Mid-anterior chest with the same radiating patterns.
Signs and symptoms	Dyspnea, nausea, signs of indigestion (e.g., burping), profuse sweating.	Nausea and vomiting, fear, diaphoresis, pounding heart, palpitations (possible).

Any patient who calls the medical office complaining of chest pain must be examined immediately. The office should have an established protocol for handling these calls. The physician needs to be consulted to decide whether the patient should be directed to the nearest emergency room, whether emergency medical services should be dispatched, or whether the patient should come directly to the office. This is not a decision that medical assistants should make.

10

Table 10-2

Comparison of Diabetic Coma and Insulin Shock

	Diabetic Coma	Insulin Shock
Onset	Gradual	Sudden
Skin	Flushed, dry	Pale, moist
Tongue	Dry or furred	Moist
Breath	Smell of acetone	No smell
Thirst	Intense	Absent
Respiration	Deep	Shallow
Vomiting	Common	Rare
Pulse	Rapid, feeble	Rapid, bounding
Urine	Glucose and acetone present	No glucose or acetone
Blood glucose	Elevated (>200 mg/dL)	Subnormal (20 to 50 mg/dL)
Blood pressure	Low	Normal
Abdominal pain	Common, often acute	Absent

10

BOX 10-1

Emergency Care for Bleeding Wounds

Gloves are available for your protection in an office situation. Avoid exposure to blood or body fluids in a non-
medical situation.

- Control the bleeding by the method most appropriate
  for the situation:
  1. Direct pressure on the wound using sterile, nonadher-
     ent gauze in an office situation, or using cloth as clean
     as possible when sterile supplies are not available.
  2. Pressure against a pressure point proximal to the
     wound. (Review pressure points to recall them in-
     stantly in an emergency.)
- After applying pressure, assess the situation and the patient. Assess pulse, temperature, and sensation beyond
  the injury.
- Raise the site above the heart, if practical, to help control both bleeding and pain.
- If a body part is amputated, save the severed part by
  double bagging and covering with ice. Transport the
  part with the patient as quickly as possible.
- If bleeding involves an impaled object, do not remove
  the object. Immobilize the patient and the object for
  transport.
- Transport the patient to the nearest emergency room for
  assessment and treatment.
- Transport your observations and any pertinent information with the patient.

10

WARNING!

*Do not remove saturated pressure dressings. Removing dressings dis-
rupts the clotting process and renews bleeding. Reinforce dressings without disturbing the site.*

BOX 10-2

Emergency Care for Fractures

- Assume that an injured limb is fractured until proven otherwise and splint accordingly.
- Assess the situation and the patient. Assess and record pulse, temperature, and sensation beyond the injury.
- As nearly as possible, splint an injured limb without altering the position.
- Protect the site from further injury by handling it as little as possible.
- Include the joints above and below the injury in the splint to ensure that the area is immobilized.
- Transport to the nearest emergency room as quickly as possible for assessment and treatment.
- Transport your observations and any pertinent information with the patient.

10

BOX 10-3

Emergency Care for Burns

- If necessary, assess the situation for danger to you, and then remove the source of the burn.
- As needed, assess the patient for response, airway, and pulse.
- Wrap the patient in a clean, dry sheet if the burn is extensive. Cover small areas with nonadherent gauze, if available.
- Administer oxygen, if available.
- Keep the patient warm and transport as quickly as possible.
- Transport your observations and any pertinent information with the patient.

Medication Administration

The easiest and most common route of medication administration is also the most acceptable to patients.

Procedure 11-1

Administering Oral Medications

1. Assemble this equipment:
   - Medication
   - Medication tray
   - Disposable calibrated cup
   - Physician's instructions
   - Glass of water

2. Follow these Standard Precautions.

3. Select the medication. Compare the label with the physician's instructions. Check the expiration date. Check the label three times: when taking it from the shelf, while pouring, and when returning it to the shelf.
   Avoids administering outdated or incorrect medication

4. Calculate the correct dosage to be given.

5. Remove the cap from the container, touching only the outside of the lid.
   Prevents contaminating the lid

6. Remove the correct dose of medication from the container.

  a. For solid medications:

  (1) Pour the capsule or tablet into the bottle cap to prevent contamination of the cap and the medication.

  (2) Transfer the medication to a disposable cup without touching the inside of the cup or medication.

  b. For liquid medications:

  (1) Open the bottle lid and place it on a flat surface with the open end facing up to prevent contamination of the inside of the cap.

  (2) Palm the label to prevent liquids from dripping onto the label and obscuring the writing.

  (3) With the opposite hand, place the thumbnail at the correct calibration on the cup. Holding the cup at eye level, pour the medication.

  (4) Read the level at the lowest level of the meniscus, the curved surface of the medication in the container. The lowest level of the meniscus gives the proper amount of medication.

7. Greet and identify the patient. Explain the procedure. Ask the patient about medication allergies that may not be noted on the chart.
Provides information about allergies not documented

8. Give the medication to the patient.

9. Give the patient a glass of water for swallowing the medication unless contraindicated.
Assists swallowing

10. Remain with the patient to be sure that all of the medication is swallowed. Observe for any unusual reactions and report them to the physician. Record any unusual reactions on the patient's chart.
Ensures that medication has been taken; documents adverse reactions

11. Thank the patient and give appropriate instructions.

12. Wash your hands.

Procedure Notes:

WARNING!

· If the dosage requires that a scored tablet be broken, use a gauze square for breaking. Never break the tablet using bare hands.
· Never crush enteric tablets.
· Never open time-release capsules.
· Keep all medications out of the reach of children.

You Need to Know:

* Water is contraindicated when giving medications intended for local effects, such as cough syrup and lozenges, or when giving buccal or sublingual medications, which are absorbed locally for a systemic effect and must not be swallowed.
* If the patient has trouble swallowing, a large swallow of water before taking the pill or capsule may moisten the oral mucosa and make swallowing easier. Drinking through a straw or bottle with a narrow neck may make solid forms of medication easier to swallow

Instruct the Patient or Caregiver to:

* Take medications only as prescribed, and complete the course as recommended by the physician
* Take the most important medication first
* Drink a full glass of water unless contraindicated
* Sit with both feet on the floor if taking medications at night, and drink a full glass of water to prevent choking
* Never share medications with family members
* Never crush a tablet or open a capsule without checking first with the office or pharmacist
* Check with the office before stopping a medication or adding other medications

BOX 11-1

The Seven Rights of Medication Administration

1. Right patient
2. Right time and frequency
3. Right dose
4. Right route of administration
5. Right drug
6. Right technique
7. Right documentation

BOX 11-2

Dosage Calculation Formulas

- Ratio/proportion:

Dose on hand (DH):known quantity (KQ)

$\qquad$ = dose desired (DD):unknown quantity (UQ)

- Multiply the extremes (DH $\times$ UQ). Multiply the means (KQ $\times$ DD). Divide the product of the means by the product of the extremes to arrive at the dosage.
- Formula:

$$\frac{\text{Dosage desired}}{\text{dosage on hand}} \times \text{quantity} \times \left(\frac{\text{DD}}{\text{DH}} \times Q = X \right)$$

- Body surface area:

$$\frac{\text{BSA in m}^2 \times \text{adult dose}}{1.7} = \text{child's dose}$$

BOX 11-2

Dosage Calculation Formulas—cont'd

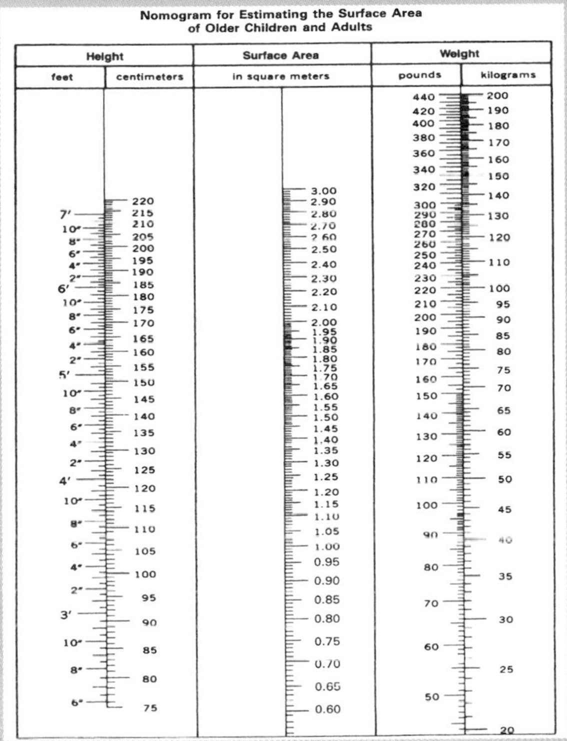

Nomogram for Estimating the Surface Area
of Older Children and Adults

Figure 11-2-1. To determine the surface area of the patient, draw a straight line between the point representing the height on the left vertical scale and the point representing the weight on the right vertical scale. The point at which this line intersects the middle vertical scale represents the patient's surface area in square meters. (Used with permission of Ross Products Division, Abbott Laboratories, Inc., Columbus, Ohio.)

Document on the Patient's Chart:

- Date and time
- Medication name
- Dose
- Route
- Reactions to medication as indicated
- Patient education and instructions
- Your signature

10/14/2004	Ampicillin 125 mg PO given stat as
12:45 PM	ordered. NKA.
	—T. Jones, RMA

II

Medications affected by gastrointestinal enzymes may be given by the sublingual or buccal routes.

Procedure 11-2

Administering Sublingual or Buccal Medication

1. Assemble this equipment:
   - Medication
   - Medication tray
   - Disposable cup
   - Physician's orders

2. through **8.** Follow steps 1 through 7 as described in Procedure 11-1: Administering Oral Medications.

9. Administer the medication.

   a. For sublingual medications, have the patient place the medication under the tongue.

   b. For buccal medications, have the patient place the medication between the cheek and gum.

10. Remain with the patient to be sure that the medication is not swallowed and is allowed to dissolve completely. Do not allow the patient to ingest any food or water until the medication is completely absorbed.
Ensures that medication has been taken properly with no adverse effects

11. Thank the patient and give appropriate instructions.

12. Wash your hands.

Procedure Notes:

WARNING!

Keep all medications out of the reach of children.

You Need to Know:

- If the patient's mouth is dry, moistening with a large swallow of water before administering the medication facilitates absorption.
- The most common sublingual medication given in the office is nitroglycerin (NTG) for chest pain.
- Observe the patient for unusual reactions to medications, and report any reactions to the physician.

Instruct the Patient to:

- Retain the medication in position and not eat or drink anything until the medication is completely absorbed
- Sit before taking NTG, because the medication causes blood pressure to decrease with vasodilation and may cause the patient to faint
- Never hold an NTG tablet in her hand; perspiration and warmth may cause it to dissolve

Document on the Patient's Chart:

- Date and time
- Medication name
- Dose
- Route
- Reactions to the medication as indicated
- Patient education and instructions
- Your signature

EXAMPLE

9/9/2004	BP: 200/120 (L), lying 198/120 (L)
4:00 PM	sitting. Procardia 30 mg/SL as
	ordered.
	—B. Wright, CMA

II

How should you prepare for an injection to decrease the risk of pain or infection for a patient?

Procedure 11-3

Preparing an Injection

1. Assemble this equipment:
   - Medication
   - Medication tray
   - Antiseptic wipes
   - Appropriate-sized needle and syringe
   - Physician's instructions
2. Follow these Standard Precautions.

3. Select the proper medication. Check the expiration date, and check the medication three times: when taking it

from the shelf, while drawing it up, and when returning it to the shelf.

Helps ensure accuracy and avoids administering outdated medication; provides for safe administration of medication

4. Calculate the correct dosage to be given.

5. Open the sterile syringe and needle package(s). Assemble if necessary.

6. Check to make sure the needle is firmly attached to the syringe by grasping the needle at the hub and turning it clockwise onto the syringe held in the other hand. Remove the needle guard.

Secures needle to avoid detachment during the procedure

7. Withdraw the correct amount of medication from the ampule or vial.

   a. From an ampule:

      (1) With the fingertips of one hand, tap the stem of the ampule lightly to remove any medication in or above the narrow neck.

      (2) Place a piece of gauze around the ampule neck to protect your fingers from broken glass. Grasp the gauze and ampule firmly with your fingers. Snap the stem off the ampule with a quick downward movement of the gauze. Be sure to aim the break away from your face. Set the ampule top aside to discard.

      (3) Insert the needle lumen below the level of the medication. Withdraw the medication by pulling back on the plunger of the syringe without letting the needle touch the nonsterile broken edge of the ampule to avoid contaminating the needle. Withdraw the desired amount of medication; set the ampule aside to dispose of properly.

      (4) If there are air bubbles in the syringe, hold it vertically with the needle uppermost and tap the barrel gently with your fingertips until the air bubbles rise to the top. Draw back on the plunger to admit a small amount of air, then gently push the plunger

forward to eject all of the air in the syringe. Do not eject any of the medication if only the required dosage has been drawn up.

b. From a vial:

(1) Cleanse the rubber stopper of the vial with the antiseptic wipe to avoid introducing microorganisms into the medication.

(2) Pull back on the plunger to aspirate an amount of air equal to the amount of medication to be removed from the vial.

(3) Insert the needle through the cleansed center of the stopper and above the level of the medication to prevent foam or bubbles from forming in the medication. Inject the air from the syringe into the vial to avoid forming a vacuum in the vial, which would make withdrawal of the medication difficult.

(4) Invert the vial, holding the syringe at eye level. Aspirate the desired amount of medication into the syringe.

(5) Remove any air bubbles in the medication within the syringe by gently tapping with your fingertips on the barrel of the syringe held vertically. Remove any air remaining in the syringe by slowly pushing the plunger. Doing this allows the air to flow back into the vial to maintain the equalized pressure.

8. Carefully recap the needle.
Protects sterility

9. Place the syringe with the medication on the medication tray with the physician's instructions. Place an antiseptic wipe on the tray for administering the medication. You are now ready to proceed with administering the specific type of injection ordered by the physician.

Procedure Notes:

You Need to Know:

- Needles and syringes are available preassembled in a package, or they may be purchased separately and assembled as needed.
- Breaking the neck of an ampule may result in almost microscopic shards of glass that may fall into the medication within the ampule. Special needle adapters are available with filters to guard against the possibility of aspirating these minute glass particles into the medication to be administered. The adapter needle is discarded after drawing up the medication, and the appropriate-sized needle for the situation is then attached to the syringe for the administration of the medication.

Is your patient allergic or sensitive to particular substances?

Procedure 11-4

Administering an Intradermal Injection

1. Assemble this equipment:
   - Medication
   - Medication tray
   - Antiseptic wipe
   - Appropriate-sized needle and syringe (generally a ⅜-inch 26- to 28-gauge needle on a tuberculin syringe to administer 0.1 to 0.2 mL)
   - Physician's instructions

2. Follow these Standard Precautions.

3. Prepare the injection according to the steps in Procedure 11-3: Preparing an Injection.

4. Greet and identify the patient. Explain the procedure. Ask the patient about medication allergies that might not be noted on the chart.
   Prevents errors; eases anxiety and ensures compliance; provides information about allergies not noted on the chart

5. Select the appropriate site for the injection. Recommended sites are the anterior forearm and the middle

11

of the back. Make sure the entire site is exposed for safety and accuracy.

6. Prepare the site by cleansing with an antiseptic wipe. Use a circular motion starting at the injection site and working outward. Do not touch the site after cleaning. If the site is grossly contaminated, wash it first with soap and water, then clean it with an antiseptic wipe.
Removes microorganisms from area; prevents bringing microorganisms back to area

7. Put on gloves.
Protects against potential exposure to blood or body fluid

8. Remove the needle guard. Using your nondominant hand, pull the patient's skin taut.
Allows needle to enter skin with less resistance; secures patient against movement

9. With the bevel of the needle facing up, insert the needle at a 10° to 15° angle into the upper layer of the skin (Figure 11-1). When correctly placed for an intradermal injection, the needle is slightly visible below the surface of the skin. The upward-facing bevel allows a wheal to form; a downward-facing bevel injects into lower tissues. It is not necessary to aspirate when performing an intradermal injection.
Ensures that penetration occurs within the dermal layer

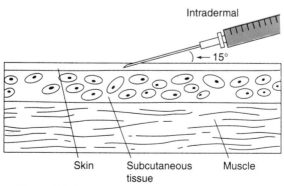

Figure 11-1. Angle of insertion for intradermal injection.

10. Release the skin held in the nondominant hand and secure the needle hub with the thumb and forefinger. Inject the medication slowly by depressing the plunger. A wheal forms as the medication enters the dermal layer of the skin. Hold the syringe steady for proper administration.

Reduces discomfort; prevents medication being pressed into tissues or out of wheal

11. Remove the needle from the skin at the same angle at which it was inserted. Gently hold an antiseptic wipe over the site as the needle is withdrawn. Do not press or massage the site.

Reduces discomfort; prevents medication being pressed into tissues or out of wheal

12. Dispose of the syringe and the needle in the approved container. Do not recap the needle. The sharps container should be placed where you will have easy access to it after administration of an injection.

Reduces risk of accidental needle stick

13. Caution the patient not to massage the site.

Avoids distributing medication into tissues

14. Remove gloves and wash your hands.

15. Remain with the patient after the administration of an intradermal injection to observe for any unusual reactions. Note: If the patient experiences any unusual reactions, notify the physician immediately.

16. Depending on the type of skin test administered, the length of time required for the body tissues to react, and the policies of the medical office, perform one of the following:

a. Read the test results. Inspect and palpate the site for the presence and amount of induration.

b. Tell the patient when (date and time) to return to the office to have the results read.

c. Instruct the patient to read the results at home and call you with his or her report. Make sure the patient understands the instructions. Have the patient repeat the instructions if necessary.

Administering an Intradermal Injection

Document on the Patient's Chart:

- Date and time
- Medication name
- Dose
- Location of injection
- Any observed reactions to medication
- Patient education and instructions for returning or reading results
- Your signature

EXAMPLE

11/9/2004	Allergy testing x14 across scapular
10:20 AM	area. Dr. Gray assessed area for re-
	actions. To RTO 11/12/2004 to begin
	immune therapy for allergies.
	—P. Ng, CMA

Procedure Notes:

WARNING!

Maintain a current and completely furnished emergency tray or cart in all sites, with special emphasis at sites that administer allergy tests or immune therapy.

You Need to Know:

- If the patient experiences any unusual reactions, notify the physician immediately; many offices require that the patient wait about 30 minutes after an injection to check for allergic reactions

Instruct the Patient or Caregiver to:

- Either return as directed for assessment of the site or read the results and report at the prescribed time

Which injection route may be used when medication requires rapid absorption?

Procedure 11-5

Administering an Intramuscular Injection

1. Assemble this equipment:
   - Medication
   - Medication tray
   - Antiseptic wipe
   - Appropriate-sized needle and syringe (generally a 1- to 2-inch, 20- to 23-gauge needle and a regular 2- to 5-mL syringe for the injection of up to 3 mL per site)
   - Physician's instructions

2. Follow these Standard Precautions.

3. Prepare the injection according to the steps in Procedure 11-3: Preparing an Injection.

4. Greet and identify the patient. Explain the procedure. Ask the patient about medication allergies that may not be noted on the chart.
   Provides information about allergies not noted on the chart

5. Select the appropriate site for the injection (see Figures 11-2 through 11-6) and the appropriate syringe.
   Avoids major nerves and blood vessels

6. Prepare the site by cleansing with an antiseptic wipe. Use a circular motion starting at the injection site and working outward. Do not touch the site after cleaning. If the site is grossly contaminated, wash it first with soap and water, then clean it with an antiseptic wipe.
   Reduces number of microorganisms

7. Put on gloves.
   Prevents potential exposure to blood or body fluids

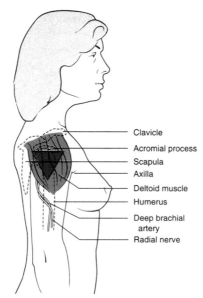

Clavicle
Acromial process
Scapula
Axilla
Deltoid muscle
Humerus
Deep brachial artery
Radial nerve

Figure 11-2. The deltoid muscle site for intramuscular injections is located by palpating the lower edge of the acromial process. At the midpoint, in line with the axilla on the lateral aspect of the upper arm, a triangle is formed.

8. Remove the needle guard. Pull the skin taut over the injection site using the nondominant hand.
Allows easier insertion of the needle; ensures that the needle enters muscle tissue

9. Hold the syringe like a dart. Using a quick, firm motion, insert the needle at a 90° angle to the skin (Figure 11-7).
Reduces discomfort, with 90° angle ensuring that medication is injected into muscle tissue

10. With the thumb and forefinger of the nondominant hand at the hub of the needle, hold the syringe steady and pull back slightly on the plunger with the dominant

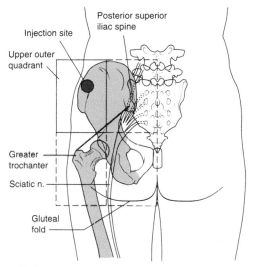

Figure 11-3. The dorsogluteal site for administering an intramuscular injection is lateral and slightly superior to the midpoint of a line drawn from the trochanter to the posterior superior iliac spine. Correct identification of this site minimizes the possibility of accidentally damaging the sciatic nerve.

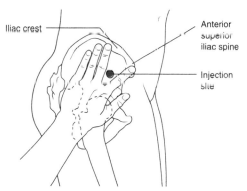

Figure 11-4. The ventrogluteal site is located by placing the palm on the greater trochanter and the index finger toward the anterior superior iliac spine. The middle finger is then spread posteriorly away from the index finger as far as possible. A "V" triangle is formed by this maneuver. The injection is made in the middle of the triangle.

hand. If blood appears in the syringe, you must prepare a new injection and repeat the previous steps.
Avoids discomfort; prevents injecting into vessel

11. Slowly inject the medication by steadily depressing the plunger of the syringe.
Prevents discomfort and tissue damage

12. Place an antiseptic wipe over the injection site. Remove the needle quickly and at the same angle at which it was inserted.
Reduces patient discomfort; prevents tissue movement when needle is withdrawn

11

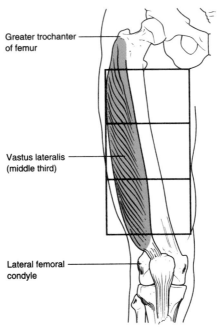

Greater trochanter of femur

Vastus lateralis (middle third)

Lateral femoral condyle

Figure 11-5. The vastus lateralis site for intramuscular injections is identified by dividing the thigh into thirds horizontally and vertically. The injection is given in the outer middle third.

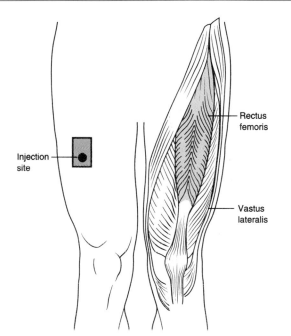

Figure 11-6. The rectus femoris site for intramuscular injections is used only when other sites are contraindicated.

13. Properly dispose of the needle and syringe in an approved sharps container. Do not recap the needle. The sharps container should be placed where you will have easy access to it after the injection has been administered.

    Reduces risk of accidental needle stick

14. Gently massage the injection site with an antiseptic wipe. Apply pressure to the site and cover with an adhesive bandage if needed.

    Distributes medication into tissue for better absorption

15. Remove gloves and wash your hands.

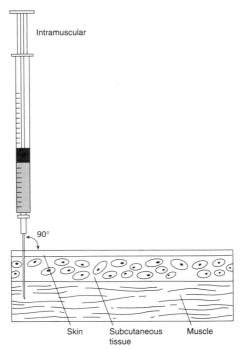

Figure 11-7. Angle of insertion for intramuscular injection.

16. Remain with the patient to observe for any unusual reactions. Assist the patient off of the examination table if necessary.

Assesses for reaction to drug effects; promotes patient safety

17. Thank the patient and give appropriate instructions.

Procedure Notes:

Document on the Patient's Chart:

- Date and time
- Medication name
- Dose
- Location of injection
- Any observed reactions to the medication
- Patient complaints or concerns
- Patient education and instructions
- Your signature

EXAMPLE

2/28/2004	PCN 200,000 u IM (L) DG as
2:25 PM	ordered. NKA.
	—M. Turner, RMA

II

You Need to Know:

- Patients with meager muscle mass may require that you grasp the muscle and "bunch" it to ensure that the medication is inserted as deeply into the area as possible.
- Carefully assess areas of repeated injections for tissue damage. If the patient is to receive frequent injections, maintain an injection chart for the patient record to document a rotation pattern to avoid overuse of a specific site.

Intramuscular Injection Using the Z-Track Method

How can you prevent a backward flow of medication that might stain or irritate upper skin layers?

Procedure 11-6

Administering an Intramuscular Injection Using the Z-Track Method

1. Assemble this equipment:
   - Medication
   - Medication tray
   - Antiseptic wipe
   - Appropriate-sized needle and syringe
   - Physician's orders

2. Follow these Standard Precautions.

3. Prepare the injection according to the steps in Procedure 11-3: Preparing an Injection.

4. Greet and identify the patient. Explain the procedure. Ask the patient about medication allergies that may not be noted on the chart.
   Provides information about allergies not noted on the chart

5. Select the appropriate site for the injection (refer to Figures 11-3 through 11-6) and the appropriate syringe.
   Note: The deltoid site does not work well for the Z-track method.
   Avoids major nerves and blood vessels

6. Prepare the site by cleansing with an antiseptic wipe. Use a circular motion starting at the injection site and working outward. Do not touch the site after cleaning. If the site is grossly contaminated, wash it first with soap and water, then clean it with an antiseptic wipe.
   Reduces the number of microorganisms

7. Put on gloves.
   Prevents potential exposure to blood or body fluids

8. Remove the needle guard. Rather than pulling the skin taut or grasping the tissue as for an intramuscular injection, pull the top layer of skin to the side and hold it with the nondominant hand.

   Seals puncture route when layers of tissue slide back to proper alignment

9. Insert the needle to the hub at a 90° angle in a quick, dart-like motion.

10. Hold the skin layer at the proper angle with the side of the hand, and grasp the needle hub or barrel with the thumb and forefinger. Aspirate by withdrawing the plunger slightly. If no blood appears, push the plunger in slowly and steadily. Count to 10 before withdrawing the needle.

    Allows time for absorption to begin

11. Cover the area with an antiseptic wipe. Withdraw the needle and release the skin. Most Z-track injections must not be massaged to avoid forcing the medication into upper tissues. Check the medication manufacturer's guidelines.

12. Properly dispose of the needle and syringe in an approved sharps container. Do not recap the needle. The sharps container should be placed where you will have easy access to it after the injection has been administered.

    Reduces risk of accidental needle stick

13. Remove gloves and wash hands.

14. Remain with the patient to observe for any unusual reactions.

    Allows time for body's reaction to drug effects

15. Thank the patient and give appropriate instructions.

Procedure Notes:

Document on the Patient's Chart:

- Date and time
- Medication name
- Dose
- Location of injection
- Any observed reactions to the medication
- Patient complaints or concerns
- Patient education and instructions
- Your signature

EXAMPLE

11/4/2004	Imferon 150 mg IM Z-track (R) DG
11:15 AM	as ordered. NKA.
	—S. Fowler, CMA

You Need to Know:

- The ventrogluteal, vastus lateralis, and dorsogluteal sites work well for the Z-track method; the deltoid site does not.

What steps should you follow for a subcutaneous injection to provide a slow, sustained release of medication?

Procedure 11-7

Administering a Subcutaneous Injection

1. Assemble this equipment:
   - Medication
   - Medication tray
   - Antiseptic wipe
   - Appropriate-sized needle and syringe, generally a ½- to ⅜-inch, 24- to 28-gauge needle on a regular 2- to 3-mL syringe or tuberculin syringe
   - Physician's order

2. Follow these Standard Precautions.

3. Prepare the injection according to the steps in Procedure 11-3: Preparing an Injection.

4. Greet and identify the patient. Explain the procedure. Ask the patient about medication allergies that may not be noted on the chart.
Provides information about allergies not noted on the chart

5. Select the appropriate site for the injection. The upper arm, thigh, back, and abdomen are common sites for subcutaneous injections. The entire site must be exposed for accuracy and safety.
Prevents errors in site identification

6. Prepare the site by cleansing with an antiseptic wipe. Use a circular motion starting at the injection site and working outward. Do not touch the site after cleaning. If the site is grossly contaminated, wash it first with soap and water, then clean it with an antiseptic wipe.
Removes microorganisms

7. Put on gloves.
Prevents potential exposure to blood or body fluid

8. Remove the needle guard. Using the nondominant hand, hold the skin surrounding the injection site in a cushion fashion.
Holds skin up and away from muscle to ensure entrance into subcutaneous tissues

9. With a firm motion, insert the needle into the tissue at a 45° angle to the skin (Figure 11-8). Hold the barrel between the thumb and index finger of the dominant hand, and insert the needle up to the hub into the tissue.
Causes less pain; ensures that medication is inserted into the proper tissue

10. Remove your nondominant hand from the skin.
Prevents injection into compressed tissue

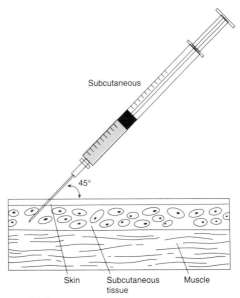

Figure 11-8. Angle of insertion for subcutaneous injection.

11. With the thumb and forefinger of the nondominant hand on the hub of the needle, hold the syringe steady and pull back on the plunger slightly. If blood appears in the syringe, a vessel has been entered. If this occurs, prepare a new injection and repeat steps 5 through 11.
Prevents patient discomfort; avoids possibility of injecting into vessel

12. Inject the medication slowly and steadily by depressing the plunger.
Avoids discomfort and tissue damage

13. Place an antiseptic wipe over the injection site and remove the needle at the same angle at which it was injected.
Reduces discomfort; prevents tissue movement when the needle is withdrawn

14. Properly dispose of the syringe and needle into an approved sharps container. Do not recap the needle. The sharps container should be placed where you will have easy access to it after giving the injection.
    Reduces risk of accidental needle stick

15. Gently massage the injection site with the antiseptic wipe. Apply pressure to the site and cover with an adhesive bandage if needed.
    Distributes medication into tissues

16. Remove your gloves and wash your hands.

17. Remain with the patient to observe for any unusual reactions. If the patient experiences any unusual reactions, notify the physician immediately.

18. Thank the patient and give appropriate instructions.

Procedure Notes:

11

WARNING!

Maintain a current and completely furnished emergency tray in all sites, with special emphasis at sites that administer allergy testing or immune therapy.

You Need to Know:

- A patient who has received an injection for allergy desensitization must remain in the office for at least 30 minutes to be observed for a reaction. Carefully assess areas of repeated injections for tissue damage.
- Heparin, which is sometimes given subcutaneously, is not massaged because it may cause excessive bleeding into the site.
- If the patient is to receive frequent injections, maintain an injection chart to document a rotation pattern to avoid overuse of a specific site.

Document on the Patient's Chart:

- Date and time
- Medication name
- Dose
- Location of injection
- Any observed reactions to the medication
- Patient education and instructions
- Your signature

EXAMPLE

9/14/2004	0.5 mL of Vial A allergy medication
9:30 AM	SQ (L) upper posterior arm. Pt.
	displayed no erythema or other
	symptoms at 30 minutes. Pt. d/c
	to return for continuing series
	9/16/2004.
	—J. Krauter, RMA

Does your patient have active or previous tuberculosis infection?

Procedure 11-8

Administering a Tine or Mantoux Test

1. Assemble this equipment:
   - Tuberculin syringe with $\frac{3}{8}$- to $\frac{1}{2}$-inch, 26- to 27-gauge needle with 0.1 mL purified protein derivative (PPD) or Tine application
   - Millimeter ruler
   - Acetone wipe or alcohol wipe

2. Follow these Standard Precautions.

3. For the Tine test, obtain the Tine applicator. For the Mantoux test, prepare the injection according to the steps in Procedure 11-3: Preparing an Injection.

4. Greet and identify the patient. Explain the procedure.

5. Assess the area of the forearm about 4 inches below the antecubital area.
Ensures an appropriate, lesion-free site

6. Clean the area with outward, circular strokes with the acetone wipe. Allow to dry.
Removes microorganisms from the site; prevents inoculation with antiseptic

7. Put on gloves.
Prevents potential exposure to blood or body fluid

8. Grasp the forearm with the nondominant hand to stretch the skin, to secure the site, and to make it easier to pierce the skin.

    a. For the Mantoux test, follow steps 9 through 12 of Procedure 11-4: Administering an Intradermal Injection.
    Inserts PPD into intradermal layer of skin

    b. For the Tine test, uncap the tester and press it into the skin. Hold for 1 to 2 seconds, release the tension on the skin, and remove the tester.
    Pierces skin and introduces PPD into intradermal layer

9. Do not massage the site in either method. Cover the site gently and briefly with an alcohol wipe, but do not press or wipe.
Prevents pressing testing material into lower skin layers or along injection line

10. Properly care for or dispose of equipment and supplies. Remove gloves and wash your hands.

11. Advise the patient regarding returning for evaluation of the test, or give instructions regarding the evaluation card to be completed in 48 to 72 hours and returned by mail.
Provides documentation of results

Document on the Patient's Chart:
- Date and time
- Medication name
- Dose
- Location of injection
- Any observed reactions to the medication
- Patient education and instructions for returning or reading results
- Your signature

EXAMPLE

4/19/2004	Mantoux test with PPD 0.1 mL ID
2:45 PM	(L) anterior forearm. Pt. instructed
	to return 4-21-2004 for assess-
	ment of test. Pt. verbalized under-
	standing of instructions.
	—A. Wang, CMA

Procedure Notes:

You Need to Know:
- Alcohol, rather than acetone, may be used if it is allowed to dry completely to avoid diluting the medication.
- If the patient is to return for evaluation of the test, read the results in a good light with the arm slightly flexed. Palpate from the outside area to the center of induration and measure using a millimeter ruler. Disregard erythema and measure only the area of induration.

Instruct the Patient or Caregiver to:
- Either return as directed for assessment of the site or read the results and report at the prescribed time

Need to wash the patient's eye? Follow these steps to ensure the patient's safety.

Procedure 11-9

Irrigating the Eye

1. Assemble this equipment:
   - Small sterile basin
   - Towels
   - Emesis basin
   - Sterile irrigating solution at about 100°F (37°C to 38°C)
   - Sterile syringe (bulb or plunger)
   - Tissues

2. Follow these Standard Precautions.

3. Greet and identify the patient. Explain the procedure.

4. Position the patient comfortably, either sitting with head tilted with the affected eye downward or lying with the affected eye downward.
   Reduces risk of contaminating the unaffected eye

5. Drape the patient with a protective barrier to avoid wetting the clothing.

6. Have the patient hold the emesis basin against the upper cheek near the eye with the towel under the basin. Glove now. With clean gauze, wipe from the inner canthus outward to remove debris from the lashes.
   Reduces risk of exposure to body fluid; prevents lash debris from washing into eye

7. Separate the lids with the thumb and forefinger of the nondominant hand. The dominant hand holding the syringe with solution may be lightly supported on the bridge of the patient's nose parallel to the eye to steady the hand.

8. Gently irrigate from the inner to the outer canthus, holding the syringe 1 inch above the eye. Use gentle

pressure and do not touch the eye. The physician's order determines the period of time required for the irrigation and the type of solution to be used.

Avoids washing pathogens into lacrimal punctum; reduces risk of touching eye and causing discomfort

9. Use tissue to wipe away any excess solution from the patient's face.

10. Properly dispose of equipment or sanitize as recommended and remove gloves. Wash your hands.

11. Thank the patient and give appropriate instructions.

Encourages positive attitude about the office and physician

Procedure Notes:

II

You Need to Know:

- Make sure the preparation is for ophthalmic purposes. Solutions used for the eye must be sterile and formulated for ophthalmic use, and they should be just above body temperature to avoid patient discomfort.
- If both eyes are to be treated, use separate equipment for each to avoid cross-contamination.
- Eye irrigations can be performed using a Morgan lens, which consists of a plastic applicator that is placed directly on the eyeball (similar to a contact lens). An attachment to the lens connects to an irrigating solution, which runs in and irrigates the eye. Before using a Morgan lens, carefully read the manufacturer's instructions.
- If the patient experiences pain during the irrigation, stop the procedure and notify the physician. Anesthetic drops may need to be applied before the treatment can continue.

Instruct the Patient or Caregiver to:

- Always position the head with the affected eye downward to avoid washing contaminants into the unaffected eye
- Discontinue treatment and contact the office immediately if the patient experiences pain during treatment
- Prevent entry of foreign objects and other injuries to the eyes by wearing goggles during procedures or activities that might result in splashes, splatters, sprays, or flying objects striking the face

Document on the Patient's Chart:

- Date and time
- Medication or type of solution
- Amount of irrigation (optional for situation)
- Length of time of irrigation
- Which eye (OD, OS, OU)
- Patient complaints or concerns
- Patient education and instructions
- Your signature

EXAMPLE

10/31/2004	CC: c/o burning OU after splashing
1:30 PM	laundry detergent into eyes. OU
	red, teary. Dr. Burns notified—
	irrigation with NS, OU performed,
	vision clear after irrigations, no
	further c/o burning.
	T. Roberts, CMA

How can you help protect the patient's vision while treating eye disorders?

Procedure 11-10

Instilling Ophthalmic Medications

1. Assemble this equipment:
   - Medication
   - Sterile gauze
   - Tissues
   - Physician's instructions

2. Follow these Standard Precautions.

3. Greet and identify the patient. Explain the procedure. Ask the patient about allergies not recorded in the chart.
Provides information about allergies not noted on the chart

4. Position the patient comfortably.
Facilitates treatment

5. Pull down the lower eyelid with the gauze and have the patient look upward.
Exposes the conjunctival sac to receive medication; helps prevent blinking

6. Instill the medication.

    a. Ointment: Discard the first bead of ointment. Place a thin line of ointment across the inside of the lower eyelid, moving from the inner canthus outward. Release the line of ointment by twisting slightly. Do not touch the tube to the eye.
    Discards first contaminated bead; prevents touching eye with tube; releases line of ointment

    b. Drops: Hold the dropper close to the conjunctival sac, about $\frac{1}{2}$ inch away; do not touch the patient. Release the proper number of drops into the sac. Discard any medication left in the dropper.
    Avoids contaminating remainder of multiple-dose container

7. Have the patient gently close the eyelid and roll the eye to disperse the medication.

8. Wipe away any excess medication with tissue. Instruct the patient to apply light pressure on the puncta for several minutes.
Prevents medication from running to nasolacrimal sac and duct

9. Properly care for or dispose of equipment and supplies. Clean the work area. Wash your hands.

Procedure Notes:

Document on the Patient's Chart:

* Date and time
* Patient complaints or concerns
* Medication name, including type (i.e., drops, ointment, and so on)
* Dose
* Location (i.e., OD, OS, OU)
* Patient education and instructions
* Your signature

EXAMPLE

3/22/2004	Cortisporin ophthalmic solution,
2:40 PM	2 gtt to OD as ordered. NKA.
	—C. White, RMA

WARNING!

Check the medication three times as outlined for medication administration. Medications must specify ophthalmic use. Medications formulated for purposes other than ophthalmic use may be harmful if used in the eye.

You Need to Know:

* The patient may be lying or sitting with the head tilted slightly back and positioned with the affected eye slightly downward to avoid the medication running into the unaffected eye.

Instruct the Patient or Caregiver to:

* Follow treatment regimens exactly, neither overmedicating nor undermedicating
* Maintain sterility of the medication and follow procedure as directed

Irrigating the Ear

Objects in the ear are easily flushed away with this procedure.

Procedure 11-11

Irrigating the Ear

1. Assemble this equipment:
   - Irrigation solution of the physician's choice at no more than 100°F (37°C to 38°C)
   - Basin for solution
   - Ear irrigation syringe or irrigating device
   - Waterproof barrier
   - Otoscope
   - Emesis basin or ear basin (to receive used solution)
   - Nonsterile gauze

2. Follow these Standard Precautions.

3. Greet and identify the patient. Explain the procedure.
   Prevents treatment errors; eases anxiety and promotes compliance

4. Position the patient comfortably in an erect position.

5. View the affected ear with an otoscope to locate the problem.
   - For adults: Gently pull up and slightly back to straighten the auditory canal.
   - For children: Gently pull slightly down and back to straighten the auditory canal.
   - Remove any obvious debris at the entrance of the canal before beginning the irrigation.
     Prevents washing debris further into canal

6. Drape the patient with a waterproof barrier.
   Prevents discomfort

7. Tilt the patient's head toward the affected side.
   Facilitates solution flow

8. Place the drainage basin beneath the affected ear to catch the outflow.

9. Fill the syringe or turn on the irrigating device.

10. Gently position the auricle as described above with the nondominant hand. (Refer to Figure 8-4.)
    Straightens canal for either visualization or treatment

11. With the dominant hand, place the tip of the syringe into the auditory meatus, and direct the flow of solution gently upward toward the roof of the canal.
    Avoids pressure against tympanic membrane and facilitates outflow of solution

12. Continue irrigating for the prescribed period of time.

13. Dry the patient's external ear with gauze. Have the patient sit for a while with the affected ear downward to drain the solution.
    Provides for patient comfort

14. Inspect the ear with the otoscope to determine the results.
    Observes for success of treatment

15. Properly care for or dispose of equipment and supplies. Clean the work area. Wash your hands.

Procedure Notes:

WARNING!

If the tympanic membrane appears to be perforated, do not irrigate without checking with the physician; solution may be forced into the middle ear through the perforation.

You Need to Know:

- Ear irrigations are not usually painful, but the flow of the solution may be uncomfortable. The patient may be more cooperative if this is understood.

Instruct the Patient or Caregiver to:

- Avoid using any object to clean the ear canal because this may drive cerumen or foreign bodies deeper into the canal
- Caution young children about placing small objects into the ear; small objects may require surgical removal

Document on the Patient's Chart:

- Date and time
- Type of solution or medication
- Which ear (AD, AS, AU)
- Description of outflow, if used to remove debris or foreign objects
- Patient complaints or concerns
- Patient education and instructions
- Your signature

EXAMPLE

6/7/2004	CC: 30-month-old "tugging" on AS
12:30 PM	after "putting kernel of corn" into
	ear canal x20 min. ago. Dr. Rogers
	notified. AS irrigated with 500 mL
	NS, return clear with x1 kernel of
	corn.
	—R. Lowe, CMA

Instilling a topical ear medication? Use this simple procedure.

Procedure 11-12

Instilling Otic Medication

1. Assemble this equipment:
   - Medication with dropper
   - Cotton balls
   - Physician's order

2. Follow these Standard Precautions.

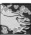

3. Greet and identify the patient. Explain the procedure.

4. Have the patient seated with the affected ear tilted upward.
   Allows medication to flow through canal to area of concern

5. Draw up the ordered amount of medication.

6. Grasp auricle as follows:
   • For adults: Pull the auricle slightly up and back to straighten the S-shaped canal.
   • For children: Pull the auricle slightly down and back to straighten the S-shaped canal.

7. Insert the tip of the dropper without touching the patient's skin, and let the medication flow along the side of the canal.
   Avoids contaminating dropper; allows medication to flow gently to avoid patient discomfort

8. Have the patient sit or lie with the affected ear upward for a short while.
   Allows medication to rest against the tympanic membrane for as long as possible

9. If the medication is to be retained, insert the cotton ball slightly into the external auditory meatus without force.
   Keeps medication in canal; avoids patient discomfort

10. Thank the patient and give appropriate instructions.

11. Properly care for or dispose of equipment and supplies. Clean the work area. Wash your hands.

Procedure Notes:

WARNING!

· *If the tympanic membrane appears to be perforated, do not instill anything into the ear canal without checking with the physician; medication may be forced into the middle ear through the perforation.*
· *Check the medication three times as specified for medication administration. The label must specify otic preparation.*

Document on the Patient's Chart:

- Date and time
- Medication name
- Dose
- Location (i.e., AD, AS, AU)
- Patient complaints or concerns
- Patient education and instructions
- Your signature

EXAMPLE

2/19/2004	Debrox otic solution x5 gtts AD as
5:30 PM	ordered.
	—W. Graham, CMA

11

You Need to Know:

- Ear instillations are not usually painful, but the flow of the solution may be uncomfortable. The patient may be more cooperative if this is understood.

Instruct the Patient or Caregiver to:

- Complete all prescribed antibiotic ear medications, either oral or topical, even though symptoms may subside; the infection may still be present even though the patient is asymptomatic

How do you administer medications formulated for the nasal passages?

Procedure 11-13

Instilling Nasal Medication

1. Assemble this equipment:
   - Medication drops or spray
   - Tissues
   - Physician's instructions

2. Follow these Standard Precautions.

3. Greet and identify the patient. Explain the procedure. Ask the patient about allergies not documented.
Prevents errors; eases anxiety and ensures compliance; provides information about allergies not noted on the chart

4. Position the patient in a comfortable recumbent position. Extend the patient's head beyond the edge of the examination table or place a pillow under the patient's shoulders. Support the patient's neck to avoid strain as the head is tilted back.
Allows medication to reach upper nasal passages

5. Put on gloves now.
Prevents contact with potentially hazardous body fluid

6. Administer the medication.

    a. For nose drops: Hold the dropper upright just above each nostril and drop the medication one drop at a time without touching the nares. Keep the patient in the recumbent position for 5 minutes.
Avoids contaminating dropper; allows medication to reach upper nasal passages

    b. For nasal spray: Have the patient sit. Place the tip of the dispenser at the naris opening without touching the patient's skin or nasal tissues, and spray as the patient takes a deep breath.
Allows medication to reach upper nasal passages

7. With tissues, wipe away excess medication from the patient's skin.
Avoids patient discomfort

8. Thank the patient and give appropriate instructions.

9. Properly care for or dispose of equipment and supplies. Clean the work area. Remove gloves. Wash your hands.

Procedure Notes:

Document on the Patient's Chart:

- Date and time
- Medication, including form (such as drops or spray)
- Dose
- Location (which nostril, or naris)
- Patient complaints or concerns
- Patient education and instructions
- Your signature

EXAMPLE

11/2/2004	CC: c/o dry, itchy nares bilaterally.
10:45 AM	Saline spray to both nares as
	ordered.
	—C. Simon, RMA

You Need to Know:

- Check the medication three times as specified for medication administration. Preparations for use in the nasal passages must be formulated for these surfaces.
- Nasal instillations may be uncomfortable but should not be painful.

Instruct the Patient or Caregiver to:

- Guard against children placing small objects in the nose
- Prevent rebound phenomenon that may cause addiction to nasal products if used more frequently or for longer periods than prescribed

Dermal medications are applied directly to the skin to produce local effects.

Procedure 11-14

Applying Topical Medications

1. Assemble this equipment:
   - Medication
   - Medication tray

- Physician's order
- Washing solution (optional)
- Tongue blade
- Large cotton-tipped swab
- Dressing, bandage, tape (optional)

2. Follow these Standard Precautions.

  (optional)

3. Greet and identify the patient. Explain the procedure. Ask the patient about medication allergies that might not be noted on the chart.
   Provides information about allergies not documented

4. Assess the area to record observations regarding the condition of the skin.
   Aids in accurate documentation before obscuring site with medication

5. Put on gloves, in most instances.
   Prevents contact with lesions or absorption of medication if medication is touched

6. If the area is soiled, clean the skin according to the steps for skin preparation.
   Ensures clean skin

7. If old medication remains in the area from a previous treatment, remove it by the same procedure.
   Prevents applying new medication over old medication

8. If the lesion requires a dressing and bandage, apply the medication to the dressing using a tongue blade.
   Reduces patient discomfort

9. If the medication is to be applied directly to the area, lightly spread it with a tongue blade or a large cotton-tipped swab, working from the center of the area outward.
   Prevents returning microorganisms to site of concern

10. Use clean technique or medical asepsis if there are no open lesions. Use no-touch technique or surgical asepsis if the skin is broken.

11. Bandage if necessary.
    Protects wound

Document on the Patient's Chart:

- Date and time
- Medication name
- Dose
- Location of application
- Any observed reactions to the medication
- Patient education and instructions
- Your signature

	EXAMPLE
7/19/2004	Delacort applied to x3 lesions on
4:35 PM	(R) anterior forearm as directed.
	—T. Cruz, CMA

II

12. Thank the patient and give appropriate instructions. Assist as needed.

13. Clean the treatment room and dispose of equipment and supplies appropriately. Wash your hands.

Procedure Notes:

You Need to Know:

- Avoid touching the medication with your hands, because you may absorb unneeded medication.
- Assess the patient's or caregiver's level of comprehension for application at home and report your concerns.

Instruct the Patient or Caregiver to:

- Gently remove a previous application before applying a new dose; use soap and water unless contraindicated
- Observe for unusual reactions to the medication and report the reaction to the physician

When medication is ordered for a slow, steady absorption, follow these steps.

Procedure 11-15

Applying Transdermal Medications

1. Assemble this equipment:
   • Medications
   • Medication tray
   • Physician's order

2. Follow these Standard Precautions.

     (optional)

3. Greet and identify the patient. Explain the procedure. Ask the patient about medication allergies that may not be noted on the chart.
   Provides information about allergies not previously documented

4. Select the site for administration and perform any necessary skin preparation. The sites are usually the upper arm, the chest or back surface, or behind the ear; these should be rotated. Ensure that the skin is dry, clean, and free of any irritation. Do not shave areas with excessive hair; trim the hair closely with scissors.
   Ensures appropriate absorption, prevents abrading skin to avoid rapid medication absorption

5. You may glove at this point. If there is a patch already in place, remove it carefully. If you choose not to glove, do not touch the inside of the patch to avoid absorbing any remaining medication. Discard the used patch. Inspect the site for irritation.
   Prevents absorption into your skin

6. Open the medication package by pulling the two sides apart. Do not touch the area of medication.

7. Apply the medicated patch to the patient's skin following the manufacturer's directions. Press the adhesive edges down firmly all around, starting at the center and

Document on the Patient's Chart:

- Date and time
- Medication name
- Dose
- Location of patch
- Any observed reactions to the medication
- Patient education and instructions
- Your signature

EXAMPLE

09/06/2004	Transdermal NTG patch applied to
8:30 AM	(L) anterior chest as ordered. BP
	178/88 (L).
	—R. Evans, RMA

pressing outward. If the edges do not stick, fasten with paper tape.

Eliminates air spaces and ensures close contact with skin

8. Thank the patient and give appropriate instructions.

9. Wash your hands.

Procedure Notes:

You Need to Know:

- To avoid skin irritation, always rotate sites.
- Always remove the old patch before applying the new to avoid an overdose of medication.

Instruct the Patient or Caregiver Regarding:

- Proper technique for application and safety of administration
- Safety measures for preventing contact by anyone other than the patient

Surgical Procedures

Do you need to remove hair and surface contaminants? Follow these steps.

Procedure 12-1

Hair Removal and Skin Preparation

1. Assemble this equipment:
   - Shaving cream or lotion
   - New razor
   - Gauze or cotton balls and warm rinse water
   - Antiseptic solution
   - Sponge forceps
     Or
   - Commercially packaged skin preparation kit
   Note: If the skin is not to be shaved and is not grossly soiled, you need only antiseptic solution and gauze or cotton balls, or antiseptic wipes.

2. Follow these Standard Precautions.

3. Greet and identify the patient. Explain the procedure and answer any questions.

4. Prepare the patient's skin.

   a. If the patient's skin is to be shaved, apply shaving cream or soapy lather to the area to be shaved. Pull the skin taut and shave by pulling the razor across the skin in the direction of hair growth. Repeat this procedure until all hair is removed from the operative area. Rinse and pat the shaved area thoroughly dry using a gauze square.

Allows close shave; reduces risk of abrasions

b. If the patient's skin is not to be shaved, rinse away any soapy solution used for general cleaning, and dry the skin before applying antiseptic solution to avoid diluting the antiseptic.

5. Apply antiseptic solution of the physician's choice to the skin surrounding the operative area using sterile gauze sponges, sterile cotton balls, or antiseptic wipes. With the gauze or cotton ball grasped in the sterile sponge forceps, wipe the skin in any of the pictured patterns, starting at the operative site and working outward (Figure 12-1). Discard each sponge after a complete sweep has been made.

Prevents wound contamination by microorganisms brought from surrounding skin

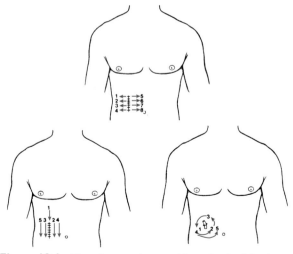

Figure 12-1. Clean the wound outward from the site following any of the numbered patterns.

Document on the Patient's Chart:

- Date and time
- Area of skin preparation
- Any lesions, open areas, or rashes in the skin preparation area
- Patient education and instructions
- Your signature

EXAMPLE

9/12/2004	CC: excision of mole (R) shoulder
4:30 PM	today as scheduled. Skin shaved,
	prepped with Betadine solution.
	—A. Bolin, RMA

6. With dry, sterile gauze sponges grasped in the sponge forceps, pat the area thoroughly dry. In some instances, the area may be allowed to air dry.
Prevents wetting drape, which could wick contaminants to operative site

7. Instruct the patient not to touch or cover the prepared area.
Avoids contaminating operative site

8. Drape the prepared area for the procedure, or cover it with sterile drapes if the procedure is delayed for a short time. Longer delays may require reapplication of the antiseptic solution.
Prevents contaminating operative site

Procedure Notes:

Assisting With Excisional Surgery

You Need to Know:

- If the area to be prepared is large or circles are not appropriate, wipe straight outward from the operative site, using each sponge once before it is discarded, and repeat the procedure until the entire area has been thoroughly cleaned. At no time should a wipe that has passed over the skin be returned to the already cleaned area or to the antiseptic solution.
- Use care when shaving or preparing around moles, warts, or other skin irregularities. Nicks and cuts to these structures may delay healing and can open areas of the integument to the entrance of pathogens.
- The time spent preparing the skin may be used to assess the patient's response to the procedure to be performed. Use this time to elicit questions and concerns and to answer those questions that are within your scope of practice; refer all other questions to the physician.

12 What steps should you follow to assist the physician with an excision of tissue?

Procedure 12-2

Assisting With Excisional Surgery

1. Assemble this equipment:
   At the side
   - Sterile gloves
   - Local anesthetic
   - Antiseptic wipes
   - Adhesive tape
   - Bandages
   - Specimen container with completed laboratory request
   On the field
   - Basin for solutions
   - Gauze sponges and cotton balls
   - Sterile drape
   - Dissecting scissors or iris scissors
   - Scalpel blade and handle of physician's choice
   - Mosquito forceps
   - Needle holder

- Suture and needle of physician's choice (Note: These may be at the side if physician prefers the site be numbed before gloving.)

2. Follow these Standard Precautions.

3. Greet and identify the patient. Explain the procedure and answer any questions.

4. Set up a sterile field on a surgical stand with at-the-side equipment close at hand. Cover the field with a sterile drape if necessary until the physician arrives.

5. Position the patient appropriately.
   Increases patient comfort and provides access to surgical site

6. Prepare the site following Procedure 12-1: Hair Removal and Skin Preparation.
   Protects against wound contamination from surface microorganisms

7. Watch closely for opportunities to assist the physician and to comfort the patient (i.e., putting on sterile gloves and passing instruments to the physician from the field, adding supplies, and so forth).
   Allows for procedural flow with fewer complications

8. At the end of the procedure, dress the wound using the procedure for applying a sterile dressing (Procedure 12-7).
   Protects wound from contamination

9. Assist the patient from the table and offer to help with clothing as needed. Thank the patient and give appropriate instructions.
   Prevents falls and increases safety; encourages positive attitude about office and physician

10. Clean the examining room in preparation for the next patient. Discard all disposables in appropriate biohazard containers. Return unused reusable items to their proper places. Wash your hands.
    Prevents spread of pathogens; reduces waste

Document on the Patient's Chart:

- Date and time
- Location of procedure
- Type of specimen and routing procedure
- Type of dressing
- Patient complaints or concerns
- Patient education and instructions
- Your signature

EXAMPLE

3/26/2004	CC: removal of nevus (L) periorbital
10:30 AM	ridge scheduled, specimen to lab,
	dry sterile dressing applied to
	surgical site. Verbal and written
	post-op instructions given
	regarding wound care. RTO in
	7 days for suture removal.
	—J. Cohen, CMA

Procedure Notes:

You Need to Know:

- If the lesion is to be referred to pathology for analysis, you will be required to assist with the specimen container during the procedure.
- Some physicians prefer that the site be cleaned and made ready by an assistant; others prefer doing it themselves after gloving, using the supplies on the field. In all instances, the physician's preference takes precedence over any outlined procedure.

12

Suppurative lesions may require an incision to relieve pressure and speed the healing process.

Procedure 12-3

Assisting With Incision and Drainage (I & D)

1. Assemble this equipment:

   At the side
   - Sterile gloves
   - Local anesthetic
   - Antiseptic wipes
   - Adhesive tape
   - Sterile dressing packs
   - Packing gauze
   - Bandages
   - If the wound is to be cultured, a culture tube is also included at the side

   On the field
   - Basin
   - Sterile cotton balls or gauze
   - Antiseptic solution
   - Sterile drape
   - Syringes and needles for local anesthetic (Note: These should be at the side if the physician prefers the site to numb before gloving)
   - Commercial I & D set or scalpel, dissecting scissors or operating scissors, hemostats, tissue forceps, 4 × 4 gauze sponges, probe (optional)

2. Follow these Standard Precautions.

3. Greet and identify the patient. Explain the procedure and answer any questions.

4. Set up a sterile field on a surgical stand with at-the-side equipment close at hand. Cover the field with a sterile drape if necessary until the physician arrives.

5. Position the patient appropriately.
   Increases patient comfort and provides access to surgical site

12

6. Cleanse the site with sterile antiseptic solution in the manner described for skin preparation (Procedure 12-1).
Reduces surface microorganisms

7. Watch closely for opportunities to assist the physician and to comfort the patient (i.e., putting on sterile gloves and passing instruments to the physician from the field, adding supplies, and so forth).
Allows for procedural flow with fewer complications

8. At the end of the procedure, dress the wound using the procedure for applying a sterile dressing (Procedure 12-7).
Protects wound from contamination

9. Assist the patient from the table and offer to help with clothing as needed. Thank the patient and give appropriate instructions.
Prevents falls and increases safety

10. Clean the examining room in preparation for the next patient. Discard all disposables in appropriate biohazard containers. Return unused reusable items to their proper places. Wash your hands.
Reduces waste

Procedure Notes:

12

You Need to Know:

- Exudate from infected lesions is an especially high risk for contamination. As always, observe Standard Precautions to avoid the spread of pathogens.

Instruct the Patient or Caregiver to:

- Practice good hygiene to avoid recurrence
- Avoid tight clothing and occlusive cosmetics; both are known to contribute to abscess formation
- Avoid squeezing lesions to prevent pressing contamination into surrounding tissues
- Isolate wash cloth and towel until no longer infected to avoid passing infection through the family

Document on the Patient's Chart:

- Date and time
- Location of procedure
- Type of specimen (i.e., wound culture) and routing procedure
- Patient's temperature or other vital signs, if indicated by the infectious process or patient complaints
- Any complications with procedure
- Patient education and instructions
- Your signature

EXAMPLE

3/15/2004	I & D of abscess (L) hand, third digit
11:00 AM	per Dr. Moore. Dry sterile dressing
	and tubular bandage applied post-
	op. Pt. instructed to return for
	wound check in 3 days. Written and
	verbal post-op instructions given to
	pt.—verbalized understanding.
	—P. Abbe, RMA

12

- Launder clothing and linens separately
- Discard dressings, bandages, and supplies in impervious bags

How should you assist in a lumbar puncture to diagnose central nervous system disorders?

Procedure 12-4

Assisting With a Lumbar Puncture

1. Assemble this equipment:
   At the side
   - Adhesive bandages
   - Sterile gloves (may be on the field or at the side)

- Skin preparation supplies
- Blood pressure cuff (if Queckenstedt test is to be performed)
- Completed laboratory slips for cerebrospinal fluid

On the field

- Local anesthetic and syringe (Note: These should be on the field if the physician prefers to administer the anesthesia from the sterile field)
- Lumbar needle with a stylet (physician specifies gauge and length)
- Sterile gloves for the physician
- Gauze sponges
- Specimen tubes for transport
- Spinal fluid manometer with a three-way stopcock adapted (if cerebrospinal fluid pressure is to be measured)
- Fenestrated drape
- Sterile drape
- Antiseptic

Note: Commercial lumbar puncture surgical trays contain all needed supplies

2. Follow these Standard Precautions.

3. Greet and identify the patient. Explain the procedure. Tell the patient that the puncture will be made below the level of the spinal cord and should present no danger to the patient. Warn the patient not to move during the procedure. Tell the patient that the area will be numbed but that pressure may still be felt after the local anesthetic is administered.

4. Check that the consent form is signed and posted on the chart.
   Adheres to legal requirement for written consent for invasive procedures

5. Have the patient void.
   Prevents one source of discomfort during procedure

6. Direct the patient to disrobe and put on a gown with
the opening in the back.
Exposes site for procedure

7. Determine and record the vital signs.
Provides baseline vital signs

8. When the physician is ready, open the field (follow the
steps described for opening sterile surgical packs and
assist with the initial preparations) (Procedure 7-9).

9. Prepare the skin if this is not done as part of the sterile
preparation. Many physicians prefer to prepare the
skin using a sterile forceps after gloving. If this is the
preferred procedure, you may be required to add sterile solutions to the field (follow the steps for adding
sterile solutions to a sterile field) (Procedure 7-10).

10. Assist as needed with administration of the anesthetic.

11. Assist the patient into the appropriate position.

   a. For the side-lying position: Stand in front and help
   by holding the knees and top shoulder. Have the
   patient move so that his back is close to the edge of
   the table.

   b. For the forward-leaning, supported position: Stand
   in front and rest your hands on the patient's shoulders as a reminder to remain still. Have the patient
   breathe slowly and deeply.
   *Positions patient to widen space between vertebrae to allow
   entrance of needle; helps prevent movement during procedure*

12. Throughout the procedure, observe the patient closely
for signs such as dyspnea or cyanosis. Monitor the
pulse at intervals.

13. When the physician has the needle securely in place,
help the patient to straighten slightly to ease tension
and to allow a more normal cerebrospinal fluid flow.
The physician may now use the stopcock and spinal
fluid manometer to determine the intracranial and in-
traspinal pressure.

14. If specimens are to be taken, put on gloves to receive
the potentially hazardous body fluid. Label the tubes

in sequence as you receive them. Also label them with the patient's identification and place them in biohazard bags. Be aware that the first tube may be more likely to contain contaminants.

15. If the Queckenstedt test is to be performed, you may be required to press the veins of the neck with your hands, first the right, then the left, then both sides, each for 10 seconds, while the physician measures the pressure with the stopcock and manometer. In an alternate method, the physician places a blood pressure cuff around the patient's neck before gloving for the procedure and instructs you to inflate the cuff to 22 mm Hg for 10 seconds while she measures the pressure with the manometer.

16. At the completion of the procedure, cover the site with an adhesive bandage and assist the patient to a supine position. Record the vital signs after the procedure. Note mental alertness, any leakage at the site, nausea, and vomiting. Assess lower limb mobility. The physician determines when the patient is ready to leave the examining room and the office.
Observes for complications during recovery

17. Route the specimens as required.
Ensures that specimens are transported properly

18. Clean the room and care for or dispose of the equipment as needed. Wash your hands.

Procedure Notes:

You Need to Know:

- Most offices stock the equipment in a purchased disposable tray or a site-prepared setup.
- Before beginning, assess the lumbar region. If the skin is very hairy, it may be necessary to shave the skin before the procedure. Strict asepsis must be observed to reduce the risk of introducing microorganisms into the nervous system.

Document on the Patient's Chart:

- Date and time
- Vital signs before and after procedure; include the temperature, particularly if the procedure is for a fever of unknown origin (FUO)
- Patient's tolerance of the procedure and complaints or concerns
- Patient education and instructions
- Your signature

EXAMPLE

2/12/2004	Pt. positioned and draped for lum-
8:30 AM	bar puncture. T 99.2 (o) P 86, R
	18 BP 120/80 (L).
	—B. Ryan, CMA
9:00 AM	LP completed per Dr. Alexander. Pt.
	tolerated procedure well. CSF
	specimen to lab as ordered Post-
	LP VS T 98.0 (o) P 76 R 16 BP:
	114/74 (L). Pt. resting comfortably.
	—B. Ryan, CMA
9:30 AM	Pt. denies discomfort. No n/v. No
	leakage at LP site. Pt. and wife
	given verbal and written discharge
	instructions. Verbalized understand-
	ing. Pt. discharged by Dr. Alexander.
	—B. Ryan, CMA

12

Removing Staples

- Although there is little chance of damage to the cord, movement may cause the patient injury and may contaminate the field.
- The Queckenstedt test helps to determine the presence of an obstruction in the cerebrospinal fluid flow. Normally, the pressure increases and decreases rapidly during the procedure. If an obstruction is present, the increase and return to normal may be very slow or there may be no response to the external application of pressure.

Instruct the Patient to:

- Remain still throughout the procedure; movement may contaminate the field or cause the patient pain
- Breathe slowly and deeply to help in relaxation

How should you remove surgical staples?

Procedure 12-5

Removing Staples

1. Assemble this equipment:
   - Antiseptic solution or wipes
   - Gauze squares
   - Sponge forceps
   - Instrument for removing staples
   - Sterile gloves
     Or
   - Sterile, disposable, staple removal kit

2. Follow these Standard Precautions.

3. Greet and identify the patient. Explain the procedure and answer any questions.

4. If the dressing and bandages have not been removed, glove and remove them now. Dispose of dressings properly in a biohazard container. Remove the gloves and wash your hands.

5. Using the "no-touch" technique, clean the incision with antiseptic solution. Pat dry using dry, sterile

gauze sponges. While you are performing these tasks, assess the healing stage.
Helps avoid wound infection; aids in visualizing staples

6. Put on sterile gloves.
Maintains sterility

7. Gently slide the end of the staple remover under each staple to be removed. Press the handles together to lift the ends of the staple out of the skin and remove the staple (Figure 12-2).
Lifts ends free and minimizes patient discomfort

8. Place each staple on a gauze square as it is removed.
Aids in counting staples

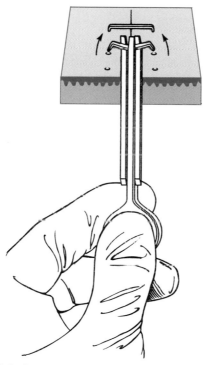

12

Figure 12-2. Slide the end of the staple remover under each staple. Press the handles together to lift the ends of the staple out of the skin.

9. Clean the site with an antiseptic solution, and if the physician has indicated to do so, cover with a sterile dressing.
   Protects as needed

10. Thank the patient and give appropriate instructions.

11. Properly care for or dispose of all equipment and supplies. Clean the work area. Remove gloves and wash your hands.

Procedure Notes:

WARNING!

Do not remove staples without an expressed order by the physician. The degree of healing should be assessed by the physician before the staples are removed.

12

You Need to Know:

- As the dressing is removed from the wound, the physician may be called to assess the healing process. The wound may need to be assessed both before and after exudate is removed.

Instruct the Patient or Caregiver to:

- Avoid tension on the site for several days after the staples are removed
- Continue wound treatments as prescribed by the physician for the recommended number of days, and report any concerns immediately
- Watch for excessive bleeding or swelling, redness, or temperature elevation
- Keep the wound clean and dry until completely healed

Document on the Patient's Chart:
- Date and time
- Location of staples
- Number of staples removed
- Any difficulty with staple removal
- Any signs or symptoms of infection
- Patient complaints or concerns
- Patient education and instructions
- Your signature

EXAMPLE

7/17/2004	Staples to RLQ of abd.
12:48 PM	×4 removed as ordered. Wound
	well-approximated, no redness or
	drainage.
	—H. Hood, CMA

12

Time for suture removal? Follow these steps.

Procedure 12-6

Removing Sutures

1. Assemble this equipment:
   - Thumb forceps
   - Suture scissors
   - Gauze
   - Antiseptic
     Or
   - Sterile, disposable, suture removal kit
2. Follow these Standard Precautions.

3. Greet and identify the patient. Explain the procedure and answer any questions.

4. If dressings have not been removed previously, glove now and remove the dressing. Properly dispose of dressings. Then clean the wound area as directed. Assess the healing stage. Remove and dispose of the soiled gloves used for the soiled dressing.
   Prevents contamination of the wound; aids in visualizing sutures

5. Open the suture removal packet using surgical asepsis, or set up the field for on-site sterile equipment. Put on sterile gloves.
   Maintains sterility

6. Note that the knots are tied in such a way that one tail of the knot is very close to the surface of the skin, while the other is closer to the area of suture that is looped over the incision.

7. Remove the sutures (Figure 12-3).

   a. Grasp the end of the knot that is closest to the skin surface and lift up, slightly and gently, away from the skin.

   b. Cut the suture below the knot as close to the skin as possible.
      Frees uncontaminated area of knot; only suture below skin is pulled through tissues

   c. Use the thumb forceps to pull the suture out of the skin with a smooth, continuous motion at a slight angle in the direction of the wound.
      Avoids tension on healing tissue

8. Place the suture on a gauze sponge. Repeat the procedure for each suture.
   Helps count number of sutures removed to compare with number inserted

9. Clean the site with an antiseptic solution and, if the physician has indicated, cover with a sterile dressing.
   Protects as needed

10. Thank the patient and give appropriate instructions.

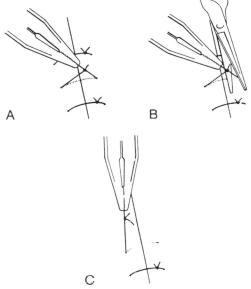

Figure 12-3. (A) With the hemostat or forceps, lift the stitch upward and away from the skin surface. This permits the blades of the scissors to slide under the stitch. **(B)** Cut the stitch near the skin. **(C)** Using the forceps, pull the freed stitch up and out.

11. Properly care for or dispose of equipment and supplies. Clean the work area. Remove gloves and wash your hands.

Procedure Notes:

WARNING!

Do not remove sutures without an expressed order by the physician. The degree of healing should be assessed by the physician before the sutures are removed.

Document on the Patient's Chart:

- Date and time
- Location of sutures
- Number of sutures removed
- Any difficulty with suture removal
- Any signs or symptoms of infection
- Patient complaints or concerns
- Patient education and instructions
- Your signature

EXAMPLE

09/15/2004	X6 sutures removed from (L) el-
9:45 AM	bow wound, edges approximated,
	no drainage.
	—J. Robertson, CMA

12

You Need to Know:

- As the dressing is removed from the wound, the physician may be called to assess the healing process. The wound may need to be assessed both before and after exudate is removed.
- Always remove sutures by pulling up and slightly toward the wound to avoid tension on the wound edges.

Instruct the Patient or Caregiver to:

- Avoid tension on the site for several days after the sutures are removed
- Continue wound treatments as prescribed by the physician for the recommended number of days, and report any concerns immediately
- Watch for excessive bleeding or swelling, redness, or temperature elevation
- Keep the wound clean and dry until completely healed

Should the wound be covered with a sterile dressing?

Procedure 12-7

Applying a Sterile Dressing

1. Assemble this equipment:
   - Sterile gloves
   - Dressings
   - Scissors
   - Appropriate bandages and tapes
   - Any medication to be applied to the dressing
   Or
   - Disposable dressing change kit

2. Follow these Standard Precautions.

3. Greet and identify the patient.

4. Ask about any tape allergies before deciding on the type of tape to use. With the size of the dressing and bandage in mind, cut or tear lengths of tape to secure the bandage. Set the tape aside in a convenient location.
   Prevents skin irritation from tape; promotes efficiency

5. Explain the procedure, and instruct the patient to remain still during the procedure and to avoid coughing, sneezing, or talking until the procedure is complete.
   Helps prevent contamination of sterile supplies and wound

6. Open the dressing pack to create a sterile field. Observe the principles of surgical asepsis. Many packets are designed to be opened by the peel-apart method.
   Ensures sterility of opened dressing

   a. If sterile gloves are to be used for the procedure, open the package of appropriate-size sterile gloves. Using sterile technique, put on the gloves (see Procedure 7-3 for applying sterile gloves).
   Avoids contamination of dressings or wound

12

b. If using a sterile transfer forceps to apply the dressing (the "no-touch" method), use sterile technique to arrange the dressing on the wound site, and do not touch the dressing or the site with your hands.
Avoids contamination of dressings or wound

7. Using the already-opened sterile dressings and principles of sterile technique, apply to the wound the number of dressings needed to properly cover and protect the wound. Be sure to carefully place sterile dressings on the wound; do not drag them over the skin into position.
Prevents contaminating dressing and wound

8. Apply the bandage so that it completely covers the sterile dressing and conforms to the patient's contours. The bandage should extend at least 1 inch beyond the border of the dressing.
Completely protects wound from outside contaminants

9. Apply the previously cut lengths of tape over the bandage in a manner that secures both bandage and dressing. Apply tape sufficiently to secure the bandage, but avoid overuse of tape. (When the wound is completely covered, you may remove your gloves, or you may prefer to keep them on during the taping. Discard them in the proper receptacle.)
Secures bandage to provide safety for patient

10. Assist the patient from the examination table.
Prevents falls and promotes patient safety

11. Properly care for or dispose of equipment and supplies. Disposable articles contaminated with blood or wound drainage require special disposal protocol. Clean the work area. Wash your hands.

12. Return reusable supplies (unopened sterile gloves or dressings, bandages, tape) to their appropriate storage areas; all others should be discarded correctly.
Prevents waste

Procedure Notes:

Document on the Patient's Chart:

- Date and time
- Location and type of dressing
- Any signs or symptoms of infection
- Presence and type of drainage
- Patient complaints or concerns
- Patient education and instructions
- Your signature

EXAMPLE

4/15/2004	Excision of sebaceous cyst (R)
12:30 PM	shoulder per Dr. Redd. Minimal
	sanguineous drainage. Dry sterile
	dressing applied to wound. Verbal
	and written instructions given to
	pt. about wound care—verbalized
	understanding.
	—C. Vasquez, CMA

12

You Need to Know:

- Before applying dressings, assess the wound for healing stages. Report your concerns to the physician.
- Clean the wound in the approved manner before applying the dressing.
- If medication is to be applied to the wound, apply it first to the dressing, then apply the dressing to the wound. By doing this, you avoid touching the wound, which might cause discomfort to the patient.
- Tape is used only to keep the dressings and bandages in place. Tape should not completely obscure the bandage, but should allow for observation of any bleeding or drainage. Too much tape can cause perspiration to dampen the dressing and compromise sterility. Tape should not obstruct blood circulation.
- Paper tape is recommended when the patient's skin is very thin and fragile, as in elderly patients.

Changing an Existing Sterile Dressing

- Provide the patient or caregiver with an approved brochure for sterile dressing changes in the home, and determine that the directives are understood.

Instruct the Patient or Caregiver to:

- Perform proper handwashing.
- Properly dispose of biohazardous material
- Recognize signs that should be reported, such as excessive redness, drainage, discomfort, and so on
- Follow office protocol for bandaging procedure

Is healing not yet complete? Should the wound still be covered?

Procedure 12-8

Changing an Existing Sterile Dressing

1. Assemble this equipment:
   - Sterile dressings and sterile gloves (for applying the new dressing)
   - Skin antiseptic solution with sterile gauze squares or sterile cotton balls, or premedicated antiseptic wipes of the physician's choice
   - Sterile basin (to receive the solution and gauze or cotton)
   - Tape, torn to appropriate lengths and set aside
     Or
   - Disposable dressing change kit

2. Follow these Standard Precautions.

3. Greet and identify the patient. Explain the procedure and answer any questions.

4. Prepare a sterile field (Procedure 7-9):

   a. If using a sterile container and solution, open the package containing the basin using sterile tech-

BOX 12-1

Bandaging Guidelines

- Observe medical asepsis. Surgical asepsis is required for dressings, but medical asepsis is appropriate for bandages.
- Keep the wound dressing and bandage dry to avoid wicking microorganisms to the site.
- Never place bandages against a wound: dressings cover the wound; bandages cover the dressing and should extend at least 1 inch beyond the dressing.
- Do not dress skin surfaces together; pad opposing surfaces to prevent tissues from adhering during healing. The entire site may be bandaged together, but should be dressed separately.
- Pad joints and bony surfaces to prevent friction.
- Bandage a part in its normal, slightly flexed position to avoid muscle strain.
- Begin the bandage distally and work proximally.
- Talk with the patient to assess the level of discomfort; adjust the bandage for comfort and security.
- When bandaging extremities, leave the fingers or toes exposed for evaluating circulation.
- Know the various techniques for wrapping bandages (see Figure 12-4).

12

nique, and use the inside of the wrapper as the sterile field for the basin.

b. Peel apart the wrappers for the gauze or cotton balls, and flip them into the basin or use sterile transfer forceps to place them in the basin (Procedure 7-11).

Avoids wound contamination

5. Prepare antiseptic solution:

a. First pour off a small amount of the solution into a waste receptacle.

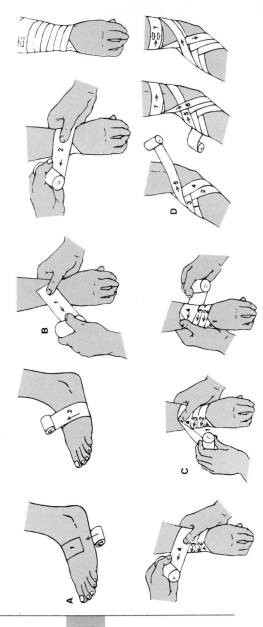

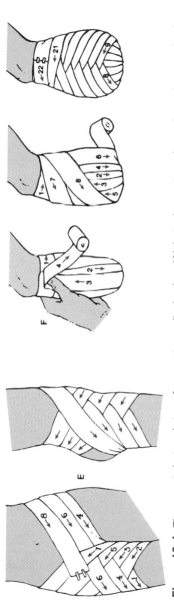

Figure 12-4. There are six basic techniques for wrapping a roller bandage. **(A)** A circular turn is used to anchor and secure a bandage when it is started and ended. It simply involves holding the free end of the rolled material in one hand and wrapping it about the area, bringing it back to the starting point. **(B)** A spiral turn partly overlaps a previous turn. The overlapping varies from one-half to three-fourths the width of the bandage. Spiral turns are used when wrapping a cylindrical part of the body such as the arm or leg. **(C)** A spiral-reverse turn is a modification of a spiral turn. The roll is reversed halfway through the turn. This works well on tapered body parts. **(D)** A figure-eight turn is best used when an area spanning a joint, such as the elbow or knee, requires bandaging. It is made by making oblique turns that alternately ascend and descend, simulating the numeral 8. **(E)** A spica turn is a variation of the figure-eight turn. It differs in that the wrap includes a portion of the trunk or chest. **(F)** The recurrent turn is made by passing the roll back and forth over the tip of a body part. Once several recurrent turns have been made, the bandage is anchored by completing the application with another basic turn such as the figure-eight. A recurrent turn is especially beneficial when wrapping the stump of an amputated limb.

12

b. Then pour the solution from the stock bottle into the sterile container on the sterile field (Procedure 7-10).
Removes possible pathogens from mouth of bottle

6. Instruct the patient not to talk, cough, sneeze, laugh, or move during the procedure.
Prevents contamination of sterile field

7. Wearing clean gloves, carefully remove the tape from the bandage by pulling it toward the wound. Cut large bandages that encircle a limb with bandage scissors, cutting on the side of the limb away from the wound. Remove the old bandage and dressing.
Prevents potential exposure to blood and body fluid; avoids tension on wound site

8. Discard the soiled dressing in a biohazard container. Do not pass it over the sterile field.
Prevents contact with hazardous material; avoids contaminating field

9. Inspect and observe the wound for degree of healing, amount and type of drainage, appearance of wound edges, and so on.
Allows evaluation of wound exudate before cleaning

10. Observing medical asepsis, remove and discard gloves.
Prevents contact with blood or body fluid

11. Put on sterile gloves. Clean the area with the antiseptic solution of the physician's choice. Clean in a circular motion from the wound site outward. If a circular motion is not appropriate for this wound, use sweeps of the antiseptic-soaked gauze from the wound outward. Discard each gauze square after a single wipe. Never return the wipe to the antiseptic solution or to the skin after one sweep across the area (Figure 12-1).
Provides clean area for wound dressing; reduces surface microorganisms

12. Replace the dressing using the procedure for sterile dressing application (Procedure 12-7).

Procedure Notes:

Document on the Patient's Chart:

- Date and time
- Location and type of dressing
- Any signs or symptoms of infection
- Presence and type of drainage
- Patient complaints or concerns
- Patient education and instructions
- Your signature

EXAMPLE

8/31/2004	CC: Sterile dressing change to ul-
1:30 PM	cerated wound on (R) heel. Mod.
	amt. of yellow purulent drainage
	noted. Dr. Carson aware. Culture
	obtained as ordered and sent to
	lab. Wound cleansed with Betadine
	solution before redressed. Pt. RTO
	in AM for dressing change.
	—T. Carter, CMA

12

WARNING!

Never pull on a dressing that does not come off easily. The healing process may be disrupted.

You Need to Know:

- If the dressing is difficult to remove because of dried wound exudate or blood, it may be soaked with sterile water or saline for a few minutes to loosen it for removing. Gently pull the edges of the dressing toward the center. If this procedure does not loosen the dressing or causes undue discomfort to the patient, notify the physician immediately.

- The physician should inspect the wound before exudate or drainage is removed. Decisions must be made regarding the healing process. If a culture is ordered, it must be taken before the wound is cleaned to ensure the most reliable test results.

Instruct the Patient or Caregiver to:

- Perform a proper handwashing
- Properly dispose of biohazardous material
- Recognize signs that should be reported, such as excessive redness, drainage, bleeding, discomfort, and so on
- Follow office protocol for bandaging procedure

Tubular gauze is quick and convenient and offers a secure and comfortable binding over dressings applied to wounds.

12

Procedure 12-9

Applying a Tubular Gauze Bandage

1. Assemble this equipment:
   - Tubular gauze
   - Applicator
   - Tape
   - Scissors

2. Follow these Standard Precautions.

3. Greet and identify the patient. Explain the procedure and answer any questions.

4. Choose the appropriate-size tubular gauze applicator and gauze width. (Manufacturers of tubular gauze supply charts with suggestions for the most appropriate size to use for various body parts.)
   Allows applicator and gauze to slip easily over body part

5. Select and cut or tear adhesive tape in lengths to secure the gauze ends.
Promotes efficiency

6. Place the gauze bandage on the applicator in the following manner:

   a. Be sure the applicator is upright (open end up) and placed on a flat surface.

   b. Pull a sufficient length of gauze from the stock box; do not cut it at this time.

   c. Open the end of the length of gauze and slide it over the upper end of the applicator; continue pushing until all of the gauze needed for this procedure is on the applicator.

   d. Cut the gauze when the required amount of gauze has been transferred to the applicator.

7. Place the applicator over the distal end of the affected part (e.g., finger, toe, leg) and begin to apply the gauze. Hold it in place as you move to step 8.
Ensures that application begins distally and wraps proximally

8. Slide the applicator containing the gauze up to the proximal end of the affected part. Turn the applicator one full turn while holding the gauze in place. Holding the gauze at the proximal end of the affected part, pull the applicator and gauze toward the distal end.
Secures bandage for application

9. Continue to hold the gauze in place. Pull the applicator 1 to 2 inches past the end of the affected part if the part is to be completely covered. In many instances, the gauze is not required to extend beyond a limb and may cover only the area around the wound.
Secures bandage at distal end; adequately covers and protects dressing

10. Turn the applicator one full turn to anchor the bandage.
Secures bandage with twist

11. Move the applicator toward the proximal part as before.
Provides a double layer of bandage for protection

12

12. Move the applicator forward about 1 inch beyond the original starting point. Anchor the bandage again by turning it as before.
Anchoring provides a secure fit.

13. Repeat the procedure until the desired coverage is obtained. The final layer should end at the proximal part of the affected area. Any extra length of gauze not needed can be cut from the applicator. Remove the applicator.
Covers the wound for protection

14. Secure the bandage in place with adhesive tape, or cut the gauze into two tails and tie them at the base of the tear. Tie the two tails around the closest proximal joint. Use adhesive tape sparingly to secure the end if not using a tie.
Secures the bandage until it must be changed

15. Thank the patient and give appropriate instructions.

16. Properly care for or dispose of equipment and supplies. Clean the work area. Wash your hands.

12

Procedure Notes:

You Need to Know:

- Before applying the dressing, assess the wound for healing. Report your concerns to the physician.
- Tubular gauze may be applied over dressings after a sterile dressing change.
- Choose an applicator slightly larger than the part to be covered. The gauze designed to fit the chosen applicator provides a secure fit.

Instruct the Patient or Caregiver to:

- Perform a proper handwashing
- Properly dispose of biohazardous material
- Recognize signs that should be reported, such as excessive redness, bleeding, drainage, discomfort, and so on
- Follow office protocol for bandaging procedure

Document on the Patient's Chart:

- Date and time
- Location and type of dressing
- Any signs or symptoms of infection
- Patient complaints or concerns
- Patient education and instructions
- Your signature

EXAMPLE

1/6/2004	CC: laceration to (R) palm
1:30 PM	occurred while cutting meat at
	home in kitchen. Wound cleansed
	with antiseptic solution. Last
	tetanus booster X 1 yr. ago.
	X 4 sutures inserted per Dr.
	Preston with no. 1-0 silk. Dry sterile
	dressing applied, tubular gauze to
	cover. Pt. to keep wound dry and el-
	evated. RTC in 3 days for recheck.
	—P. Merriwether, CMA

12

13

Specialty Procedures

Gynecologic Procedures

How can you make a patient's pelvic examination and Pap smear proceed smoothly?

Assisting With a Pelvic Examination That Includes a Pap Smear

1. Assemble this equipment:
   - Patient drape
   - Vaginal speculum, appropriate size
   - Uterine sponge forceps
   - Cotton-tipped applicators, long
   - Water-soluble lubricant
   - Direct lighting
   - Cleansing tissues or personal wipes
   - Materials for Pap smear: cervical spatula or cervical brush, glass slides, fixative solutions (spray or liquid), laboratory request form, identification label

2. Follow these Standard Precautions.

3. Label and date each slide.
   Provides proper slide identification

4. Complete the laboratory request form for Pap smear with essential information, including the date, patient's name, age, first day of last menstrual period, relevant history, physician, and your signature.
Provides information for accurate assessment of slides

5. Greet and identify the patient. Explain the procedure.

6. Ask the patient to empty her bladder, and if necessary collect a urine specimen.
Increases patient comfort; provides specimen as needed

7. Provide patient with a drape and ask her to disrobe from the waist down.
Protects patient's privacy while allowing access to pelvic region

8. When the physician enters the room, position the patient in the dorsal lithotomy position with buttocks at the bottom edge of the table.
Facilitates physician's access to pelvic region

9. Adjust the drape to cover the patient's abdomen and knees, exposing only the genitalia.
Protects patient privacy while allowing access to pelvic region

10. Adjust the light over the genitalia for maximum visibility.
Provides illumination for evaluation

11. Assist the physician with the examination by handing instruments and supplies as needed.
Increases efficiency of examination

12. Glove and hold the slides while the physician obtains the specimen and makes the smears.
Prevents exposure to biohazardous material

13. Spray each slide with fixative, or immerse each slide in a fixative solution
Preserves specimen for cytology

14. Explain to the patient that next the physician will remove the vaginal speculum and do a manual examination.
Informs patient of progress through procedure

15. Hold a basin for receiving the now-contaminated vaginal speculum. Place the speculum in a basin of soaking solution to begin sanitization.
Makes sanitization easier

13

16. Apply lubricant across the physician's two fingers.
Provides lubricant to decrease patient discomfort

17. After completion of the examination, assist the patient in sliding up to the top of the examination table.
Ensures safety

18. Assist the patient in removing both feet at the same time from the stirrups. Help the patient to remove excess lubricant by handing her a personal wipe or tissues.
Reduces strain on patient's back; increases patient comfort

19. Package the specimen for transport to the laboratory.
Provides for safe transportation or mailing to laboratory

20. Provide for privacy while the patient is dressing.
Protects privacy

21. Thank the patient. Reinforce the physician's instructions about follow-up. Address any concerns or questions.

22. Properly care for or dispose of equipment. Clean the examination room. Wash your hands.

13

Procedure Notes:

You Need to Know:

- Do not have the patient assume the examination position until the physician has entered the room. This is a difficult position to maintain, and the patient is put at a psychological disadvantage if greeting the physician in this position.
- Patients who cannot assume the dorsal lithotomy position may be examined in the semi-Fowler or Sims position.

Instruct the Patient to:

- Avoid douching or intercourse within 24 hours before a Pap smear; either may disrupt the cervical mucosa and interfere with the diagnostic results of the test
- Schedule her appointment 1 week after the last day of her menstrual period for the most accurate diagnostic test results

Document on the Patient's Chart:

- Date and time
- Patient preparation
- Patient complaints or concerns
- Patient education and instructions
- Routing of specimen
- Your signature

EXAMPLE

5/18/2004	CC: annual physical exam per Dr.
9:30 AM	Jacobs. Pap smear specimen to lab.
	Pt. Instructed verbally and in writing
	on procedure for obtaining results.
	—K. Thomas, RMA

Does the physician need to examine a patient's cervical mucosa by microscope?

13

Procedure 13-2

Assisting With Colposcopy With Cervical Biopsy

1. Assemble this equipment:
   - Setup for pelvic examination
   - Colposcope
   - Specimen container with preservative, 10% formalin
   - Sterile gloves
   - Povidone-iodine (Betadine)
   - Sanitary napkin, mini pad, or tampon
   - Silver nitrate sticks or ferric subsulfate (Monsel) solution
   - On the sterile field:
     —Cotton-tipped applicators, long, sterile
     —Normal saline solution
     —3% acetic acid or vinegar
     —Uterine dressing forceps
     —Sterile 4 × 4 gauze
     —Sterile towel

- • Sterile materials for cervical biopsy:
  —Biopsy forceps or punch
  —Uterine curet
  —Endocervical curet
  —Uterine tenaculum

2. Follow these Standard Precautions.

3. Verify that the patient has signed the consent forms, which are required for invasive procedures.
Ensures that patient is properly informed about procedure and has given informed consent

4. Check the light on the colposcope.
Ensures that equipment is functioning

5. Set up the sterile field (Procedure 7-9).
Establishes surgical asepsis for invasive procedure

6. Pour normal saline and acetic acid into their respective sterile containers (Procedure 7-10). Cover the field with a sterile drape.
Provides solutions for microscopic examination of cervix; maintains sterility

7. Greet and identify the patient. Explain the procedure. Caution the patient that there may be a sharp cramp at the time of biopsy. Have the patient disrobe from the waist down and cover with a privacy drape.

8. When the physician enters the room, position the patient in the dorsal lithotomy position.
Aids in visualizing cervix

9. If gloved to assist from the field, hand the physician the applicator immersed in normal saline, followed by the applicator immersed in acetic acid.
Acetic acid improves visualization and aids in identifying suspicious tissue

10. Hand the physician the applicator with the antiseptic (Betadine) solution.
Prevents contamination of area of biopsy

13

11. If you did not glove to assist the physician, put on nonsterile gloves before accepting the specimen.
Avoids exposure to potentially hazardous body fluids

12. Receive the tissue specimen by holding the container of 10% formalin, in which the specimen may be immersed.
Preserves specimen by immediate immersion

13. Label the specimen container with the patient's name, date, and medical record number.
Provides proper identification

14. Prepare the specimen for transport to the laboratory or pathology department.
Ensures integrity of specimen

15. Provide the physician with Monsel solution or silver nitrate sticks, if necessary.
Provides coagulation as needed

16. Explain to the patient that a small amount of bleeding may occur. Have a sanitary pad available.
Informs patient of possible concerns; provides for patient comfort

17. Thank the patient. Reinforce the physician's instructions.
Provides necessary patient instructions

13

18. Properly care for or dispose of equipment and supplies. Clean the examination room. Wash your hands.

Procedure Notes:

You Need to Know:

- Patients who cannot assume the dorsal lithotomy position may be placed in the semi-Fowler position for the procedure.

Instruct the Patient to:

- Avoid douching or intercourse within 24 hours before a colposcopy; either may disrupt the cervical mucosa and interfere with the diagnostic results of the test
- Schedule her appointment 1 week after the last day of her menstrual period for most diagnostic test results

Document on the Patient's Chart:

- Date and time
- Patient preparation
- Patient complaints or concerns
- Patient education and instructions
- Routing of specimen as needed
- Your signature

EXAMPLE

4/7/2004	Pt. positioned and draped for col-
2:00 PM	poscopy per A. Jones ARNP. Cervical
	biopsy specimen sent to laboratory.
	Minimal bleeding, no c/o discomfort.
	Verbal and written instructions
	given regarding postprocedure care.
	Verbalized understanding.
	—A. Ziegler, CMA

13

Does a patient need a contraception method that does not require oral administration? The IUD may be a good choice.

Procedure 13-3

Assisting With the Insertion of an Intrauterine Device

1. Assemble this equipment:
   - At the side
     —Setup for pelvic examination
     —Sanitary pad
     —Cleansing tissues or personal wipes

—Sterile gloves for medical assistant, or sterile transfer forceps

—Scissors

- On the sterile field
    —Uterine tenaculum

    —Uterine sound

    —Antiseptic solution (Betadine)

    —Container for solution

    —Sterile 4 × 4 gauze

    —IUD insertion kit

    —Sterile gloves for physician (possibly at the side)

2. Follow these Standard Precautions.

3. Verify that the patient has signed the consent form.
Adheres to legal requirements for informed consent for IUD insertion

4. Greet and identify the patient. Explain the procedure.

5. Have the patient disrobe from the waist down and cover with a privacy drape. Position and drape the patient in the dorsal lithotomy position, as you would for the pelvic examination.
Facilitates examination

6. Put on gloves or use sterile transfer forceps. Set up the sterile field using strict sterile technique (Procedures 7-9 and 7-11).
Reduces risk of infection

7. Pour antiseptic solution into the sterile container on the sterile field (Procedure 7-10).
Antiseptic solution reduces risk of infection.

8. Assist the physician as directed with gloving and gowning. Adjust the light source over the perineum.
Facilitates procedure

9. Open the IUD insertion kit using sterile technique. Drop the kit onto the sterile field or allow the physi

13

cian to grasp it from the opened package. The physician inserts the IUD at this point.
Maintains sterile technique

10. Have scissors available for the physician to trim the string of the IUD to just beyond the external cervical os.

11. Assist the patient back up on the table, and help her remove her legs from the stirrups.
Aids in assessing patient response to procedure; promotes patient safety

12. Provide the patient with cleansing tissues or personal wipes.
Provides for patient comfort

13. Instruct the patient on how and when to check for IUD placement.
Provides patient education

14. Have the patient check for the placement of the IUD before leaving the office.
Increases patient compliance; provides opportunity for additional patient instructions as needed

15. Offer the patient a sanitary pad for the small amounts of bleeding that may occur.
Provides for patient comfort

16. Thank the patient. Reinforce the physician's instructions regarding follow-up and side effects.

17. Properly care for or dispose of equipment and supplies. Clean the room. Wash your hands.

Procedure Notes:

You Need to Know:

- IUD insertion is usually scheduled during the menstrual period to ensure that there is no pregnancy and to facilitate insertion through a slightly dilated cervical os.

Document on the Patient's Chart:

- Date and time
- Verification of consent
- Performance of procedure
- Patient complaints or concerns
- Patient education and instructions
- Your signature

EXAMPLE

1/9/2004	Insertion of IUD per Dr. Lyons. Pt.
1:00 PM	given verbal and written instruc-
	tions on checking for placement.
	Verbalized understanding.
	—R. Jones, CMA

Instruct the Patient to:

- Check IUD placement after each menstrual period to be sure of correct position
- Report signs such as missed period, excessively heavy period, severe cramping, unusual vaginal discharge, lower abdominal pain, chills, fever, string that cannot be located, or string that feels longer
- Schedule a follow-up visit within 4 to 6 weeks, if no problems are presented

Time to remove the IUD? Follow this procedure.

Procedure 13-4

Assisting With Removal of an Intrauterine Device

1. Assemble this equipment:
   - Patient drape
   - Vaginal speculum
   - Uterine dressing forceps
   - Cleansing tissues or personal wipes
   - Sanitary pad or tampon

Assisting With Removal of an Intrauterine Device

2. Follow these Standard Precautions.

3. Greet and identify the patient. Explain the procedure.

4. Position the patient in the dorsal lithotomy position.
Facilitates visualizing string

5. Glove and assist the physician as required: adjust the light source, hand the instruments, and receive the contaminated materials on tray or basin.
Facilitates procedure; reduces exposure to hazardous material

6. Assist the patient back up on the table, and help remove her legs from the stirrups.
Protects patient from injury; provides opportunity to assess patient's response to procedure

7. Offer the patient a sanitary pad or tampon.
Provides for patient comfort

8. Thank the patient. Reinforce the physician's instructions.

9. Properly care for or dispose of equipment and supplies. Clean the examination room. Wash your hands.

Procedure Notes:

Instruct the Patient to:

- Practice alternate methods of birth control if applicable
- Avoid pregnancy until after at least one regular menstrual cycle

13

Document on the Patient's Chart:

- Date and time
- Removal of the IUD
- Patient complaints or concerns
- Patient education and instructions
- Your signature

EXAMPLE

2/12/2004	IUD removed per Dr. Williams. Pt.
10:30 AM	tolerated procedure well. Patient
	educated regarding birth control
	options.
	—A. Hood, CMA

Does a patient need a steady, predictable level of hormonal contraception?

13

Procedure 13-5

Assisting With the Insertion of a Subdermal Hormonal Implant

1. Assemble this equipment:
   - Norplant System kit
   - Sterile gloves
   - Sterile towel
   - Light source
   - Local anesthetic
   - Additional materials on sterile field:
     —Antiseptic solution
     —Sterile container for antiseptic
     —Sterile syringe (3- or 5-mL)
     —Sterile needle (1-inch, 23- to 25-gauge)
     —Sterile 4 × 4 gauze

Assisting With the Insertion of a Subdermal Implant

2. Follow these Standard Precautions.

3. Make sure the patient understands all aspects of the procedure. Verify that the patient has signed the consent form.
Adheres to legal requirements for informed consent for Norplant implantation; helps ease anxiety and increase compliance

4. Position the patient in the supine position.
Provides patient comfort; facilitates insertion of implants

5. Set up the sterile field (Procedure 7-9). Pour antiseptic solution (Procedure 7-10). Open and drop gauze, syringe, and needle onto field. Open Norplant system and drop onto field.
Provides all needed supplies

6. Cleanse top of anesthetic vial with alcohol preparation.
Reduces risk of contamination

7. Hold the anesthetic vial in the physician's preferred position while the physician aspirates anesthetic into syringe.
Maintains sterile technique

8. Assist the physician as necessary during the implant insertion.

9. Help the patient into an upright position.
Promotes patient safety

10. Thank the patient. Reinforce the physician's instructions.

11. Properly care for or dispose of equipment and supplies. Clean the room. Wash your hands.

Procedure Notes:

You Need to Know:

• Antiseptic solution can be poured into the sterile container on the field or onto sterile 4 × 4 gauze squares that remain on top of the inside of the packaging.

Document on the Patient's Chart:

- Date and time
- Location of subdermal implant
- Patient complaints or concerns
- Patient education and instructions
- Your signature

EXAMPLE

7/31/2004	Subdermal hormonal implant in-
9:45 AM	serted into inner surface of (L)
	upper arm per Dr. York. Pt. given
	discharge instruction sheet.
	—B. Brady, CMA

- The physician may prefer to administer the local anesthetic before gloving.
- Most physicians require the patient to have a urine pregnancy test before insertion of the implants.

13

Instruct the Patient or Caregiver to:

- Report signs and symptoms such as excessive bleeding, weight gain, depression, anxiety, nervousness, or breast pain

Other Specialty Procedures

The urinary catheterization procedure is considered a sterile procedure.

Procedure 13-6

Performing a Urinary Catheterization

1. Assemble this equipment:
   - Straight catheter tray that includes a no. 14 or no. 16 Fr. catheter, a sterile tray, sterile gloves, antiseptic solution, a specimen cup with a lid, lubricant, and a sterile drape

- Examination light
- Biohazard trash container

2. Follow these Standard Precautions.

3. Greet and identify the patient. Explain the procedure, answer any questions, give the patient appropriate gowning and draping materials, and have the patient disrobe from the waist down.
Explanations help ease anxiety and gain compliance.

4. Female Patients: Position the patient in the dorsal recumbent position. Carefully open the tray and place it between the legs of the patient. Adjust the examination light to allow for adequate visualization of the perineum. Apply the sterile gloves.
Adequate lighting is essential to visualize the urinary meatus.

Male Patients: Position the patient in the supine position. Carefully open the tray and place it to the side of the patient on the examination table (if there is sufficient room) or on top of the patient's thighs.

5. Female Patients: Carefully remove the sterile drape and place it under the buttocks of the patient without contaminating your sterile gloves.
Drape serves as a barrier and protects the examination table from spills.

Male Patients: Carefully remove the sterile drape and place it under the glans penis.
Drape serves as a barrier.

6. Open the antiseptic swabs and place upright inside the catheter tray. Open the lubricant and squeeze a generous amount onto the tip of the catheter while it is lying in the bottom of the tray.
Lubricant applied to the catheter allows for easier insertion into the urinary meatus.

7. Female Patients: Using the nondominant hand, carefully expose the urinary meatus by spreading the labia apart. This hand is now considered contaminated and

13

must not be moved out of position until the catheter is inside the urinary bladder.

Male Patients: Using the nondominant hand, carefully pick up the penis exposing the urinary meatus (pull back the foreskin on an uncircumcised male patient).

8. Female Patients: Cleanse the urinary meatus with the antiseptic swabs, going from top to bottom, using one swab for each side and one for the middle.

   Male Patients: Cleanse the urinary meatus with the antiseptic swabs, using one swab down each side of the meatus and one swab over the top of the meatus.

9. Using the sterile dominant hand, pick up the catheter and carefully insert the lubricated tip into the urinary meatus approximately 3 inches for female patients, 4 to 6 inches for male patients. The other end of the catheter should be left in the tray that will serve to collect the urine that is drained from the bladder.
   When urine begins to flow into the catheter tray, the catheter does not need to be inserted any further.

10. Once the urine begins to flow into the catheter tray, hold the catheter in position with the nondominant hand by moving the fingers downward, grasping the catheter. The dominant hand can then be used to direct the flow of urine into the specimen cup if a urine specimen is needed.

11. When the urine flow has slowed or stopped or an amount of 1,000 mL has been obtained, carefully remove the catheter by pulling it straight out.
    No more than 1,000 mL of urine should be removed from the bladder.

12. Wipe the perineum (female patients) or penis (male patients) carefully with the drape. Note the amount of urine in the tray by using the calibrations found on the inside of the tray. Dispose of the urine and the catheter appropriately.

13. If a urine specimen was obtained, properly label the specimen container and complete the necessary labora-

13

Document on the Patient's Chart:

- Date and time
- Procedure, including the size of catheter used, the amount of urine obtained, and the color of the urine
- If a specimen was obtained, record that it was either tested in the office (and include the results) or that it was sent to the laboratory
- Your signature

EXAMPLE

2/14/2004	Straight cath performed with no.
9:45 AM	14 Fr. catheter as ordered. 450 cc
	dark amber urine obtained.
	Specimen sent to lab for urinalysis
	and culture.
	—J. Wells, RMA

13

tory requisition. Process the specimen according to the guidelines of the laboratory.

14. Remove your gloves, wash your hands, and document the procedure.

Procedure Notes:

You Need to Know:

- If at any time before the catheterization the catheter or your gloves become unsterile, you should get another sterile tray and catheter kit.
- Removing more than 1,000 mL of urine from the bladder may cause painful urinary spasms.

Can the asthmatic patient describe exactly how much air he/she is able to bring into the lungs? With the peak flow meter, a precise measurement can be determined.

Procedure 13-7

Instructing a Patient in the Use of a Peak Flow Meter

1. Assemble this equipment:
   - Peak flow meter
   - Disposable mouthpiece
   - Chart for recording daily readings

2. Follow these Standard Precautions.

3. Greet and identify the patient. Explain the procedure.
   Prevents treatment errors; eases anxiety

4. If disposable mouthpiece is used, apply to the mouthpiece of the flow meter.

5. Slide the indicator button to the bottom of the flow meter or to zero using the markings calibrated on the outside of the flow meter.

6. Have the patient hold the peak flow meter upright, being careful not to block the opening on the back of the flow meter.
   Blocking the opening obstructs air movement

7. Instruct the patient to inhale as deeply as possible before placing the lips around the mouthpiece, forming a tight seal.
   Discourage patients from inhaling with the mouthpiece in the mouth.

8. Have the patient blow hard and fast into the mouthpiece, which will cause the indicator button to move upward. The final position of the indicator will correspond to the number of liters per minute on the scale.
   The "personal best" is used as a baseline peak flow measurement.

13

9. Repeat this procedure a total of three times. The best, or highest, reading should be recorded by the patient as his or her best and should be the number recorded on the chart.

To repeat the test, slide the indicator back to the bottom of the flow meter.

10. Thank the patient and reinforce the physician's instructions.

11. Properly care for or dispose of equipment and supplies. Clean the room. Wash your hands.

Procedure Notes:

You Need to Know:

- Many offices have patients keep the peak flow meters used for the demonstration. If your office does not have a supply of these, one should be available for demonstration and the patient should be given a prescription by the physician to obtain one from the pharmacy.
- Most peak flow meters come with a chart that gives normal predicted peak flow readings based on a person's sex, age, and height. This should be used as a guide.

Instruct the Patient or Caregiver to:

- Keep a chart of his or her best readings, done daily; on days when respirations seem difficult, the best readings can be used as a reference
- Wash the peak flow meter in warm soapy water, rinse well, and air dry; it should never be boiled

13

Document on the Patient's Chart:

- Date and time
- The procedure taught to the patient and the peak flow reading in the office
- Reinforcing of physician's instructions regarding checking and recording peak flow readings
- Your signature

EXAMPLE

11/10/2004	Pt. instructed on use of peak flow
9:15 AM	meter, given diary to record per-
	sonal best readings as ordered.
	Best reading today 450 L/min—
	no dyspnea or wheezing noted.
	—E. Cochran, CMA

13

These treatments are done to administer bronchodilators.

Procedure 13-8

Performing a Nebulized Breathing Treatment

1. Assemble this equipment:
   - Nebulizer machine
   - Disposable nebulizer setup
   - Saline for inhalation therapy
   - Medication (bronchodilator) as ordered by physician

2. Follow these Standard Precautions.

3. Greet and identify the patient. Explain the procedure.
   Prevents treatment errors; eases anxiety

4. Measure 2 to 3 mL of saline for inhalation and pour into the reservoir cup of the disposable nebulizer setup.

5. Calculate, measure, and pour the correct amount of medication into the reservoir cup with the saline.
   Follow the six rights of medication administration.

6. Assemble the reservoir cup, lid, tubing, and mouth-piece. Connect the other end of the tubing into the adapter on the machine.

7. Instruct the patient to hold the mouthpiece in the lips without biting. Also, have the patient breathe deeply during the treatment through the mouth.
   Mask setups are also available for infants and small children, who may not be able to hold the mouthpiece correctly.

8. Turn the machine on. Monitor the patient's pulse during and after the treatment.
   Bronchodilators often cause tachycardia.

9. When the reservoir cup is empty, turn off the machine.

10. Thank the patient and reinforce the physician's instructions.

11. Properly care for or dispose of equipment and supplies. Clean the room. Wash your hands.

Procedure Notes:

You Need to Know:

- Some physicians want patients to obtain a nebulizer and disposable setups for use at home. Assist the patient with obtaining these items as needed from a medical supply company.
- Bronchodilators often come prepackaged in single-dose containers for use in the office.

Instruct the Patient or Caregiver to:

- Report any increased shortness of breath or difficulty breathing during the treatment immediately

Document on the Patient's Chart:

- Date and time
- Name of the medication and dosage ordered
- Pulse rate before, during, and after the treatment
- Patient complaints or problems
- Your signature

EXAMPLE

4/28/2004	Nebulized breathing treatment
3:30 PM	with albuterol 3 mg as ordered.
	P 88, reg before treatment, 112
	during treatment, and 118 after
	treatment. No complaints during
	the treatment, stated breathing
	"much easier." Dr. Knox notified.
	—J. Briton, CMA

13

Why would a patient need a pulmonary function test?

Procedure 13-9

Pulmonary Function Testing

1. Assemble this equipment:
   - Spirometer
   - Disposable mouthpiece
   - Nose clip

2. Follow these Standard Precautions.

3. Greet and identify the patient. Explain the procedure.
   Prevents treatment errors; eases anxiety

4. Prepare the equipment, including calibrating the spirometer if necessary.
Ensures an accurate reading

5. Enter applicable data into the spirometer: patient's name, age, sex, race, height, weight, smoking status.

6. Instruct the patient to stand up and apply the nose clip.
Standing allows full expansion of the chest cavity; applying the nose clip prevents air movement from the nose, allowing a more precise test

7. Select the appropriate test (ordered by the physician) on the spirometer and, when indicated, have the patient blow hard into the mouthpiece until the spirometer indicates that the patient may stop blowing.
Patient will need much encouragement during this procedure

8. Offer feedback to the patient and recommendations for improvement. Repeat this procedure until three good maneuvers are obtained.

9. When finished, remove the nose clip, print the results, and notify the physician.

10. Thank the patient and properly care for or dispose of equipment and supplies. Clean the room. Wash your hands.

Procedure Notes:

WARNING!

The patient may get tired or dizzy during this procedure. Have a chair available close by for the patient to sit in should the need arise.

You Need to Know:

* Each spirometer may operate slightly differently depending on the manufacturer. Always read the manufacturer's instructions before using any equipment for the first time.
* If the machine cannot be calibrated or is not operating correctly, do not proceed with the test, but instead notify the physician and have the machine serviced appropriately.

Document on the Patient's Chart:

- Date and time
- Procedure and any difficulties experienced by the patient
- Location of the printed results
- Your signature

EXAMPLE

8/17/2004	PFT done, X3 readings obtained,
11:30 AM	printed results placed in the
	chart. Dr. Hart notified. No difficul-
	ties or complaints expressed dur-
	ing or after testing.
	—B. Lead, RMA

13

Instruct the Patient or Caregiver to:

- Report any increased shortness of breath, difficulty breathing, or dizziness during the procedure immediately; notify the physician before continuing

Could you use the pulse oximeter if the patient were wearing nail polish?

Procedure 13-10

Using the Pulse Oximeter

1. Assemble this equipment:
   - Pulse oximeter with sensor cable
2. Follow these Standard Precautions.

3. Greet and identify the patient. Explain the procedure.
Prevents treatment errors; eases anxiety

4. Make sure the sensor cable is securely attached to the oximeter machine.

5. Check the patient's index finger for nail polish and, if found, remove it.
Pulse oximeter reading may be inaccurate or unobtainable if nail polish is in place.

6. Turn the machine on. After the self-test, apply the sensor clip to the index finger with the cable lying on top of the posterior aspect of the hand.

7. Note the patient's pulse rate and oxygen saturation, which will appear on the digital screen.

8. Remove the sensor. Thank the patient and properly care for or dispose of equipment and supplies. Clean the room. Wash your hands.

Procedure Notes:

I3

WARNING!

A normal oxygen saturation reading should be above 95%. Notify the physician immediately if the reading is lower than this.

You Need to Know:

- Most pulse oximeter machines come with cable sensor attachments that can be clipped onto the patient's earlobe should the fingers be inaccessible.
- If a patient is having difficulty breathing, always record the respiratory rate and the skin color and warmth in addition to the oxygen saturation.
- The oxygen saturation is always recorded as a percentage.

Document on the Patient's Chart:

- Date and time
- Procedure, including the pulse rate (beats/min) and oxygen saturation as a percentage
- Your signature

EXAMPLE

10/15/2004	CC: c/o SOB, wheezing. Skin warm
8:30 AM	and dry, color pale. T 100.4 (o) P
	112, reg R 24, BP 136/88 (L). Pulse
	oximeter 93%. Dr. Lyttle notified.
	—B. Joseph, CMA

What equipment would you need to start an intravenous line?

13

Procedure 13-11

Starting an Intravenous Line

1. Assemble this equipment:
   - Intravenous (IV) catheter
   - IV solution (ordered by physician)
   - IV administration set
   - Blank label with an adhesive backing
   - IV pole
   - Supplies for venipuncture (alcohol wipes, gloves, tourniquet, gauze pads, biohazard sharps container)
   - Adhesive bandage tape, ½ inch

2. Follow these Standard Precautions.

3. Greet and identify the patient. Explain the procedure.
   Prevents treatment errors; eases anxiety

4. Attach a label to the IV solution bag that includes the patient's name, the date, and the time that the IV was prepared for use.
   Check the type of solution carefully against the physician's order; also check the expiration date on the solution bag and, if expired, do not use.

5. Hang the solution bag on the IV pole. Remove the administration set and close the roller clamp.

6. Carefully remove the cover from the end of the administration set spike and from the IV solution bag, insert the spiked end of the tubing into the IV fluid bag.

7. Squeeze the drip chamber until about $\frac{1}{2}$ full of IV fluid. Open the roller clamp, allowing IV fluid to displace any air in the tubing. Close the clamp when the tubing has filled completely with fluid.
   Leave covering over distal end of tubing during this process to avoid contaminating the tip.

8. Tear or cut two strips of tape (about 3 inches in length) to use for securing the IV catheter after insertion.
   Place the strips of tape in an easily accessible area.

9. Carefully choose a vein and perform a venipuncture using the appropriate technique (see Chapter 20). Insert the IV catheter and needle unit at a 15° to 20° angle. Observe for blood flashback into the flash chamber during the insertion of the catheter.

10. When blood is observed in the flash chamber, carefully insert the needle/catheter about $\frac{1}{4}$ inch further into the vein and stop. Slide the catheter off the needle while holding the flash chamber (on the needle) steady.

11. Advance the catheter into the vein up to the hub.
    Do not attempt to slide the needle back into the catheter once it has been removed.

12. With the needle partly occluding the lumen, release the tourniquet and obtain the distal end of the IV tubing, remove the protective covering.
    Keeping the needle partly inside the lumen prevents blood from flowing out of the catheter until the cover can be removed from the tubing.

13

13. Slide the needle completely out of the catheter and attach the end of the tubing to the end of the catheter hub. Secure the catheter with tape.

14. Adjust the roller clamp so the IV fluid is dripping into the drip chamber at a rate to be determined by the physician.

15. Secure the IV catheter and tubing with tape. Cover the insertion site of the catheter with a clear adhesive bandage according to office policy.

16. Properly care for or dispose of equipment and supplies and wash your hands.

Procedure Notes:

WARNING!

The rate at which the IV fluids are administered to the patient should be monitored carefully. Too much fluid administered over a short amount of time can cause an overload on the heart.

13

You Need to Know:

• IV catheters, or angiocatheters, come in sizes gauged like regular hypodermic needles.
• Only the physician can determine the type of IV fluids to be administered and the rate.
• The IV insertion site should be frequently assessed for any redness or swelling. If noted, the IV should be immediately discontinued and the physician alerted. If ordered, the IV can be reinserted in a different location, preferably in the other arm.

Instruct the Patient or Caregiver to:

• Report any pain or swelling at the IV insertion site immediately.

Document on the Patient's Chart:

- Date and time
- Size of the catheter used, IV solution, and rate of administration
- Your signature

EXAMPLE

2/14/2005	IV started as ordered, no. 16 an-
1:30 PM	giocatheter in (R) anterior fore-
	arm, Ringer's lactate at a keep-
	open rate. No redness or swelling
	at the site.
	—S. Schick, CMA

13 Pediatric Procedures

Head and chest measurements are important indicators of appropriate growth patterns.

Procedure 13-12

Measuring Head and Chest Circumference

1. Assemble this equipment:
   - Paper or cloth measuring tape
   - Growth chart

2. Follow these Standard Precautions.

3. Identify the patient.
   Prevents errors in treatment

4. Place the child supine on the examining table, or ask the parent to hold the child. Measure around the chest at

Document on the Patient's Chart:
- Date and time
- Head and chest measurements (HC, CC)
- Your signature

EXAMPLE

11/01/2004	CC: 6-month checkup. Head circum.
9:20 AM	41 cm. Chest 40.5 cm. Plotted on
	growth chart, placed in chart.
	—D. Winston, RMA

the nipple line, keeping the measuring tape at the same level anteriorly and posteriorly.
Ensures accurate measurement

5. Measure around the head above the eyebrows and posteriorly at the largest part of the occiput.
Ensures accurate measurement

6. Wash your hands.
Prevents spread of pathogens

Procedure Notes:

WARNING!
Never leave a child unattended on the examining table.

You Need to Know:
- If you need assistance, ask the parent or a coworker to hold the child in position.
- Childhood measurements are usually charted in the patient progress notes and graphed on a growth chart with other anthropometric measurements.
- If the head and chest growth are within normal limits, these measurements are not usually required after 12 months.

Mothers want to know "Is my baby growing as he should?"

Procedure 13-13

Measuring Length

1. Assemble this equipment:
   - Examining table with clean paper
   - Tape measure or measuring board
   - Growth chart

2. Follow these Standard Precautions.

3. Identify the patient.

4. Place the child on a firm examining table covered with clean paper. If using a measuring board, cover with clean paper.
   Provides firm, clean surface for measurement

5. Fully extend the child's body by holding the head in the midline. Grasp the knees and gently press flat onto the table. Mark the top of the head and the heel of the feet. Have the parent pick up the child or move the child away from the section used for measuring. Measure between the marks in either inches or centimeters. Read the measurement indicated on the measuring board, if this is the method used.
   Allows for full extension if infant or child assumes flexed position

6. Wash your hands.

Procedure Notes:

WARNING!

Never leave a child unattended on the examining table.

Document on the Patient's Chart:

- Date and time
- Measurement reading
- Your signature

EXAMPLE

4/12/2004	CC: 10-month well-baby checkup.
11:30 AM	Wt. 26# Length 79.5 cm T 98.8
	(T) P 100 R 22.
	—M. Gonzalez, CMA

You Need to Know:

- Children who cannot stand erect are measured in the supine position. If you need assistance, ask the parent or a coworker to hold the child in position. A foot board against the soles gives the most accurate measurement.
- Childhood measurements are usually charted in the patient progress notes and graphed on a growth chart with other anthropometric measurements.

13

Is your pediatric patient's growth within normal limits?

Procedure 13-14

Measuring Height

1. Assemble this equipment:
   - Wall-mounted measuring unit
   - Growth chart

2. Follow these Standard Precautions.

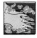

3. Identify the patient.

Document on the Patient's Chart:
- Date and time
- Measurement reading
- Your signature

EXAMPLE

	(See charting example for
	Procedure 13-13: Measuring
	Length.)

4. Explain the procedure to the parent or to the child in an age-appropriate manner.
Helps ensure cooperation

5. Remove the child's shoes. Have the child stand as tall as possible against a wall-mounted measuring unit. Make sure that the child's heels are together and that the heels, buttocks, and shoulders are against the wall unit. Have the child look straight ahead. Place the horizontal bar against the crown of the child's head to determine the measurement.
Ensures correct measurement

6. Note the measurement. Thank the child for her cooperation.

7. Wash your hands.

Procedure Notes:

13

▌**You Need to Know:**

- If the child is able to stand, height is usually the measurement of choice.
- Childhood measurements are usually charted in the patient progress notes and graphed on a growth chart with other anthropometric measurements.

Compared with other parameters, weight is one of the most important measurements for the pediatric patient.

Procedure 13-15

Weighing an Infant

 1. Assemble this equipment:
    * Infant scale
    * Protective paper for the scale
    * Growth chart

 2. Follow these Standard Precautions.

       (as needed)

 3. Identify the child.

 4. Explain the procedure to the parent or to the child in an age-appropriate manner.
    Promotes cooperation

 5. Place protective paper on the scale.
    Prevents transmission of microorganisms

 6. Balance the scale at zero.
    Ensures accuracy of measurement

 7. Place the child gently on the scale, or have the parent place the child. Infants are weighed lying down. Children who can sit may be weighed in a sitting position if this is less frightening for them. Have the parent stand in the child's view. Keep one of your hands near the child at all times.
    Provides security for child

 8. Remove an infant's diaper just before balancing the scale. Children may be weighed while wearing undergarments. Put on gloves to remove the diaper, or have the parent remove it.
    Ensures accurate reading; prevents exposure to microorganisms

13

Document on the Patient's Chart:

- Date and time
- Measurement reading
- Your signature

EXAMPLE

	(See charting example for
	Procedure 13-13: Measuring
	Length.)

9. Balance the scale quickly but carefully, moving the counterbalances to the proper places on the weight bar to exactly balance the apparatus. Have the parent pick up and soothe the child.
   Ensures accurate measurement

10. Thank the child for his cooperation.

11. Wash your hands.

Procedure Notes:

WARNING!

Wear gloves to handle diapers. Urine and feces have been implicated in the transmission of disease and require Standard Precautions.

You Need to Know:

- Childhood measurements are usually charted in the patient progress notes and graphed on a growth chart with other anthropometric measurements.
- Children who can stand may be weighed on adult scales.
- Note that cool air against the infant's skin often causes voiding.

Children's blood pressure can be measured in the same manner as that of an adult.

Procedure 13-16

Measuring Pediatric Blood Pressure

1. Assemble this equipment:
   - Stethoscope
   - Sphygmomanometer

2. Follow these Standard Precautions.

3. Select the appropriate-size cuff.
   Ensures accurate measurement

4. Identify the patient.

5. Explain the procedure to the child's parent or to the child in an age-appropriate manner. For instance, you might say, "This may squeeze your arm a little bit."
   Promotes cooperation

6. Expose the child's arm and determine the systolic pulse as described for adults.
   Identifies proper site; avoids patient discomfort or missed systolic pulse

7. Wrap the cuff around the arm 1/2 to 1 inch above the antecubitus.
   Avoids environmental noises caused by cuff touching stethoscope

8. Place the chest piece of the stethoscope at the antecubital bend. Pump the cuff about 30 mm Hg above the last pulse felt.
   Prevents discomfort while ensuring accurate measurement

9. Release the pressure 2 to 4 mm Hg per second and note the first return of the pulse. This is the systolic measurement. Note the last sound heard; this is the diastolic pressure.
   Prevents interfering with circulation or measuring inaccurately

10. Thank the child for cooperating.

11. Care for the equipment as appropriate. Wash your hands.

13

Document on the Patient's Chart:

- Date and time
- Patient complaints or concerns
- Blood pressure measurements and other vital signs as needed
- Patient or caregiver instructions and education
- Your signature

EXAMPLE

06/03/2004	CC: 9-year-old in for sports physi-
9:30 AM	cal. Ht. 4'11", Wt. 95# T 98.8 (O)
	P 84 R 22 BP 102/58 (L).
	—O. Hughes, CMA

Procedure Notes:

13

You Need to Know:

- Infants and children require a smaller cuff than adults. Choose the proper size of cuff to accurately assess the child's blood pressure.

How can you facilitate the procedure if a pediatric patient cannot lie still?

Procedure 13-17

Restraining a Child

1. Assemble this equipment:
   - Receiving blanket (if using mummy restraint)
2. Follow these Standard Precautions.

  (as needed)

3. Identify the patient.

4. Explain the purpose of the restraint to the child's parents.
Decreases parent concern regarding injury by restraint

5. Approach the child in a calm and purposeful manner. Speak softly close to the child's ear.
Reassures child and decreases anxiety

6. Restrain the child.

    a. If only physical restraint is required, stabilize the child's joints.

    b. If you are using a mummy restraint, place the child diagonally on a small receiving blanket.

    c. Wrap the right corner across the torso, covering the right arm and shoulder. Pull it snugly under the child's left arm and tuck it under the child's body (Figure 13-1A).

    d. Pull the left corner across the child's left arm and shoulder and tuck it snugly under the torso at the back so that the child's weight secures the end (Figure 13-1B). Tuck the bottom of the blanket around the child (Figure 13-1C).
    Eliminates leverage that might allow child to break from restraint

13

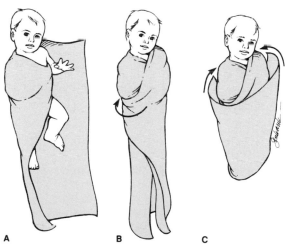

Figure 13-1. Mummy restraint.

Document on the Patient's Chart:

- Date and time
- Reason for restraint
- Procedure requiring restraints
- Type of restraints and length of time the child is restrained
- Patient complaints or concerns
- Caregiver education and instructions
- Your signature

12/14/2004	10-month-old presents with fever
10:45 AM	±102 (R) ×2 days. T 102.4 tym-
	panic P 124 R 32. Mummy re-
	straint applied for duration of ear
	exam per Dr. Carson (<5 min).
	—S. Swinson, RMA

13

7. Guard against excessive pressure on the area of the child's body that is being restrained.
   Prevents injury

8. Observe the child for any signs of respiratory distress or pain.
   Allows for adjustment of restraint or holding position to provide for comfort

9. Wash your hands.

Procedure Notes:

You Need to Know:

- Holding the closest joint stabilizes the limb. For instance, to restrain the thigh for an injection, hold the child's knee rather than the lower leg.
- For a lengthy procedure or for a larger, stronger child, it may be necessary to enlist the help of another coworker.

Is a child too young to urinate in a container on request?

Procedure 13-18

Applying a Pediatric Urine Collection Device

1. Assemble this equipment:
   - Pediatric urine collection bag
   - Personal antiseptic wipes or cotton balls
   - Completed laboratory request slip
   - Transport container

2. Follow these Standard Precautions.

3. Identify the patient.
   Prevents errors

4. Explain the procedure to the child's parent(s).
   Helps gain cooperation

5. Place the child in a supine position and ask for help from the parent as needed.
   Ensures proper attachment of collection bag; promotes compliance

6. Put on gloves.
   Prevents exposure to potentially hazardous body fluid

7. Clean the genitalia with the wipes or solution.

   a. For female patients: Cleanse front to back with separate wipes for each downward stroke on the outer labia. The last clean wipe should be between the inner labia, or labia minora.

Removes debris from area and avoids introducing microorganisms into urethra

b. For male patients: If the child is uncircumcised, retract the foreskin if possible. Cleanse the meatus in an ever-widening circle. Discard the wipe and repeat. Return the foreskin to position.

Avoids introducing microorganisms into urethra; prevents constriction of penis

8. Holding the collection device, remove the upper portion of the paper backing and press it around the mons pubis. Remove the second section and press it against the perineum. Loosely attach the diaper.

Ensures secure attachment of device; avoids soiling if child has stool

9. Give the baby fluids unless contraindicated.

Promotes urination

10. Check the diaper frequently for the specimen. When the child has voided, remove the device, clean the skin of residual adhesive, and put on a clean diaper.

Reduces skin irritation

11. Perform a routine urinalysis, or route the specimen as required. Label the specimen with the patient's name, identification number, and date.

Ensures proper specimen handling

12. Remove gloves and wash your hands.

Prevents spread of pathogens

Procedure Notes:

You Need to Know:

- Children who are old enough to understand the procedure are probably able to provide a specimen without the use of a collection device.

Document on the Patient's Chart:

- Date and time
- Application of urine collection device
- Description of urine (e.g., cloudy, bloody, clear, and so on)
- Parental or caregiver education and instructions
- Your signature

EXAMPLE

5/21/2004	5-month-old for urine specimen as
10:10 AM	ordered by Dr. Perkins. Urine collec-
	tion device applied after perineal
	prep, fluids offered. Pt. voided q. s.
	cloudy yellow urine, specimen to lab.
	—W. Maher, CMA

13

Therapeutic Procedures

Ambulatory Procedures
Does a patient require a wheelchair for assistance?

Procedure 14-1

Assisting With Wheelchair Transfer

1. Assemble this equipment:
   - Wheelchair
   - Transfer belt
   - Sliding board (optional)

2. Follow these Standard Precautions.

3. Explain to both the patient and caregiver how you can facilitate the transfer and how they both may help.
   Promotes safety; encourages patient and caregiver self-reliance

4. Organize the setting to ensure the shortest transfer distance possible and greatest ease of maneuvering. If you place the wheelchair facing the direction the patient either is facing or will need to face, you will not need to turn the patient.
   Provides for easier access

5. Align the wheelchair as close as possible to the point of transfer either at a 45° angle or parallel to the pa-

tient, preferably on the patient's strongest side, if possible. Lock the wheels and raise the foot rests.
Ensures safety; prevents rolling

6. Assist the patient into position as needed.

   a. From a vehicle: Standing at the patient's side, slide one arm under his thighs and brace his shoulders with your other arm. In one smooth movement, turn the patient in the seat until his feet are toward the ground.

   b. From the table: With one arm under his shoulders, assist him to sit. Help him to slide to the end of the table until his feet are on the table step. You may require assistance if he cannot step down.

   c. To assist the patient into the vehicle or onto the table, reverse the procedure.

7. Help her put on a transfer belt. Secure it snugly.
   Reduces risk of falling

8. Grasp the transfer belt at the back by reaching around her body, or reach under her arms and place your hands on her chest wall, not her axilla.
   Helps support upper body without causing discomfort

14

9. Have the patient grasp your shoulders, or have her reach with one hand for the far chair arm for partial support while grasping your shoulder with the other.
   Assists with leverage

10. Brace your feet apart with your right foot slightly forward. The patient's foot placement should mirror yours.
    Provides a wide base for support

11. Keep your spine straight. Flex your knees and hips and brace your knees against the patient's knees. Grasp the transfer belt or tighten your grip on the patient.
    Provides stability; prevents twisting the spine

12. Rock the patient back and forth to an agreed upon count of three. At the signal, encourage the patient to straighten her knees and hips. If she can, have her push off with her back foot.
    Provides momentum to make lifting easier

13. As you straighten, rock your weight onto your back foot and pivot the patient with her back to her destination. Keep your knees against the patient's knees. Support the patient in this position for a moment until balance is restored.
    Positions the patient for transfer; provides stability

14. Have the patient step back to the chair (table or other seat) and grasp the arms of the chair or other surface while you continue to provide stability with your knees against hers.
    Provides for greater safety

15. Shift your weight to your forward foot as the patient lowers herself to the sitting position.
    Provides momentum for sitting

16. Have her sit well back into the seat. If she is in the wheelchair, lower the foot rests and help her position her feet. If you are to push the patient, make sure her hands are in her lap.
    Promotes safety

Procedure Notes:

14

WARNING!

If the patient is too large or disabled for you to move alone, enlist help. One or both of you may be injured if you attempt to move a patient beyond your ability.

You Need to Know:

- A sliding board assists with movement if the transfer is between two relatively comparable heights. Many wheelchair arms are designed to lower for this maneuver. The board is secured between the patient's buttocks and the seat. The patient grasps the opposite chair arm and, with your assistance, slips into the chair. The procedure is easily reversed. When the transfer is complete, be sure to secure the arm into the locked position before you begin to wheel the patient.

Document on the Patient's Chart:
- Date and time
- Patient complaints or concerns
- Procedures performed, as appropriate
- Patient education and instructions
- Your signature

EXAMPLE

12/15/2004	CC: wound to (L) tibial ulcer,
3:20 PM	recheck. Sterile dressing change
	Wound pink, no undue redness,
	drainage. Pt. arrived in wheelchair.
	To RTO × 3 days for recheck and
	dressing change.
	—S. Kim, CMA

14

- It is presumed that patients who require caregiver assistance come to the office with their caregivers. Those arriving without assistance are probably proficient with minimal assistance.
- If at all possible, have the patient step out on his strongest leg. In the confines of a car or office, this may not be possible.
- Keep in mind these safety factors:
  —The patient's feet must always be on the properly positioned foot rests when the chair is in motion.
  —Back into and out of elevators.
  —Approach blind corners with caution.
  —Back down ramps to avoid having the patient pitch forward.

Instruct the Patient or Caregiver to:

- Practice good body alignment, such as flexed hips and knees, straight spine, and so forth
- Follow safety measures, such as locking wheels before transfer
- Organize the physical environment before attempting the transfer
- Perform wheelchair maintenance as directed by the manufacturer

How should you help in cast application?

Procedure 14-2

Assisting With Cast Application

1. Assemble this equipment:
   - Tubular, soft, stockinette fabric, sized to fit the limb
   - Roller padding or sheet wadding
   - Casting material, sized to fit the limb
   - Bucket of cool or tepid water
   - Plaster cast knife
   - Utility gloves for physician and for assistant

2. Follow these Standard Precautions.

3. Greet and identify the patient.

4. Assess the need for size and lengths of fabric stocking, cotton padding, and casting material.
   Ensures that material is appropriate for patient

5. At the physician's instructions, glove and begin to soak the casting material in the water. Remove the material when no more bubbles rise from the roll. Do not wring the roll; press the excess water from the roll and pull free one corner of the first layer of the roll.
   Adequately wets material without overwetting; provides physician with starting edge

6. Pass the cast knife to the physician at the completion of the procedure to trim away rough edges of the material.
   Reduces rough edges to prevent skin irritation

7. Educate the patient regarding cast care for the type of cast applied. Ask for and answer any questions.
   Prevents avoidable problems with cast care

8. If clothing has been removed for the procedure, help the patient dress because clothing may be difficult to replace after casting.

9. Care for and properly dispose of equipment and supplies. Wash your hands.

14

Procedure Notes:

You Need to Know:

- Be aware of the various types of casts that may be used (Box 14-1).

Instruct the Patient or Caregiver to:

- Be aware of the initial warmth of the drying cast; this diminishes in 20 to 30 minutes
- Keep the cast dry, if plaster; if fiberglass gets wet, dry with a hair dryer on cool-air setting
- Avoid indentations by allowing cast to dry completely before handling or propping on hard surfaces

BOX 14-1

Types of Casts

Short arm cast extends from below the elbow to mid-palm.

Long arm cast extends from the axilla to the mid-palm; the elbow is usually at a 90° angle.

Short leg cast extends from below the knee to the toes; the foot is in a natural position.

Long leg cast extends from the upper thigh to the toes; the knee is slightly flexed and the foot is in a natural position.

Walking cast may be either a short leg cast or a long leg cast; the cast is extra strong to bear weight and may include a walking heel.

Body cast encircles the trunk, usually from the axilla to the hip.

Spica cast encircles part of the trunk and one or two extremities.

Note: Body and spica casts are not usually seen in the medical office because transporting these patients as outpatients is very difficult.

14

Document on the Patient's Chart:

- Date and time
- Location of cast
- Assessment of circulation to body part
- Patient complaints or concerns
- Patient education and instructions
- Your signature

EXAMPLE

11/20/2004	Short leg cast (R) lower leg with
10:45 AM	walking heel applied by Dr. Menden-
	dez, (R) pedal pulse palpable and
	strong before and after cast appli-
	cation. (R) toes warm and pink
	with good movement.
	—A. Thompson, CMA

14

- Note that the extremities (fingers, toes) are left uncovered to check for color, swelling, numbness, and temperature; report any impairment to the physician immediately
- Report odors, staining, or undue warmth
- Prevent swelling by elevating the limb for at least 24 hours after casting and as often as possible after that time
- Never insert any object under the cast to scratch; breaks in the skin may become infected and require that the cast be removed prematurely

Is a patient immobilized by a leg cast? Axillary crutches fitted to the patient improve safety and mobility.

Procedure 14-3

Measuring a Patient for Axillary Crutches

1. Assemble this equipment:
   - Crutches with safety tips
   - Pads for the axilla and hand rests, as needed
   - Tools to tighten bolts

2. Follow these Standard Precautions.

3. Greet and identify the patient. Explain the procedure.

4. Ensure that the patient is wearing low-heeled shoes with safety soles.
   Provides proper height measurement; proper shoes help prevent falls

5. Have the patient stand erect. Support the patient as needed.
   Ensures patient safety

6. Have the patient hold the crutches naturally with the tips about 2 inches in front of and 4 to 6 inches to the side of the feet. This is called the tripod position; all crutch gaits start from this position (see Procedure 14-4: Teaching a Patient Crutch Gaits).

7. Using the tools as needed, adjust the central support in the base so that the axillary bar is about two finger-breadths below the patient's axilla. Tighten the bolts for safety when the proper height is reached.
   Allows for proper height adjustment to prevent nerve damage and increase safety

8. Adjust the handgrips by raising or lowering the bar so that the patient's elbow is at a 30° angle when the bar is gripped. Tighten bolts for safety.
   Improves safety and comfort

9. If needed, pad axillary bars and handgrips with soft material to prevent friction.
   Protects against friction and pressure; promotes patient comfort

10. Thank the patient and give appropriate instructions.

11. Properly care for or dispose of equipment and supplies. Wash your hands.

Procedure Notes:

You Need to Know:

- While using crutches, patients should wear shoes with the same heel height as worn for measuring to avoid an improper crutch fit.

Instruct the Patient or Caregiver to:

- Conduct safety checks at home for scatter rugs and cords that may cause falls
- Conduct safety checks of the crutches to ensure that bolts and wing nuts are secure and that safety tips are intact
- Be alert for axillary nerve damage that may occur if the crutches are used improperly; report numbness, tingling, or pain in the arms, hands, or fingers
  (Note: See Procedure 14-4: Teaching a Patient Crutch Gaits for documentation guidelines and charting example.)

14

Moving about with crutches takes skill and stamina. How can you teach a patient crutch gaits to increase her safety and independence?

Procedure 14-4

Teaching a Patient Crutch Gaits

1. Assemble this equipment:
   - Properly measured crutches using the preceding procedure

2. Follow these Standard Precautions.

3. Have the patient stand up from a chair. To do this, the patient holds both crutches on the affected side, then slides to the edge of the chair. The patient pushes down on the chair arm on the unaffected side, then pushes to stand. Weight should be rested on the crutches until balance is restored.

4. Ensure that the crutches are in the tripod position. The gait chosen depends on the patient's weight-bearing ability and coordination. All gaits start with the tripod position (see Procedure 14-3: Measuring a Patient for Axillary Crutches). Figure 14-1 shows diagrams of various crutch gaits.
Ensures safety and proper balance

5. Have the patient begin the appropriate gait.

    a. Three-point gait:

        (1) The affected leg can be held clear of the floor or used in concert with the crutches. Both crutches are moved forward, with the unaffected leg bearing the weight.

        (2) With the weight supported by the crutches, the unaffected, weight-bearing leg is brought past the level of the crutches. The affected leg may be supported or lightly touched down with no weight.

        (3) The steps are repeated.

    b. Two-point gait:

        (1) The right crutch and left foot are moved forward.

        (2) As these points rest, the right foot and left crutch are moved forward.

        (3) The steps are repeated.

14

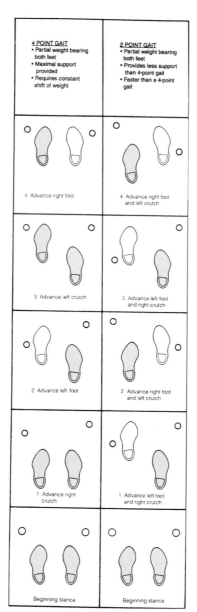

Figure 14-1. Crutch gaits.

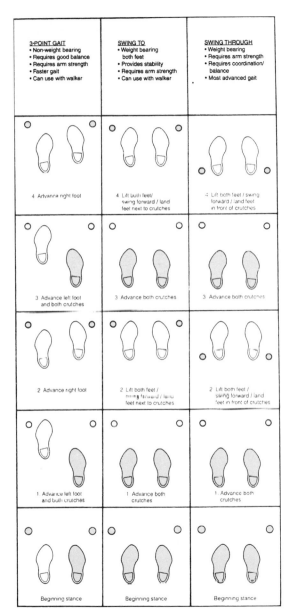

Figure 14-1. *Cont'd*

    c. Four-point gait:

        (1) The right crutch moves forward.

        (2) The left foot is moved to a position just ahead of the left crutch.

        (3) The left crutch is moved forward.

        (4) The right foot moves to a position just ahead of the right crutch.

        (5) The steps are repeated.

    d. Swing-through gait:

        (1) Both crutches are moved forward.

        (2) With the weight on the hands, the body swings through to a position ahead of the crutches.

        (3) With weight balanced on the legs, the crutches are moved ahead.

        (4) The steps are repeated.

    e. Swing-to gait: This gait may be used until the patient is ready for the swing-through gait.

        (1) Both crutches are moved forward.

        (2) With the weight on the hands, the body swings to the level of the crutches.

        (3) The steps are repeated.

  6. Thank the patient and give appropriate instructions.

Procedure Notes:

You Need to Know:

- Remind patients who require visual aids to wear them during crutch walking to reduce the risk of falls.
- Caution patients and caregivers to do a safety check of the home for scatter rugs, furniture, cords, or other safety hazards that may cause falls.

14

Document on the Patient's Chart:

- Date and time
- Type of gait taught
- Measurement of crutches to fit patient
- Patient complaints or concerns
- Patient education and instructions
- Your signature

EXAMPLE

9/15/2004	Pt. fitted for axillary crutches, el-
4:30 PM	bows flexed at 30°, two-point gait
	demonstrated with return demon-
	stration. Written and verbal in-
	structions on crutch walking given
	to pt., verbalized understanding.
	—T. Burton, RMA

14

Instruct the Patient Regarding:

- Climbing stairs:
  - —Stand close to the bottom step
  - —With weight supported on the hand rests, step up to the first step with the unaffected leg
  - —Bring the affected side and the crutches up to the step at the same time
  - —Resume balance before proceeding to the next step
  - —Remember: The good side goes up first!
- Descending stairs:
  - —Stand close to the edge of the top step
  - —Bend from the hips and knees to adjust to the height of the lower step. Do not lean forward (leaning forward may cause a fall).
  - —Carefully lower the crutches and the affected limb to the next step
  - —Next, lower the unaffected leg to the lower step and resume balance. If a handrail is available, hold both crutches in one hand and follow the steps above.
  - —Remember: The affected foot goes down first!

- Sitting:
  —Back up to the chair until you feel the edge on the backs of the legs
  —Move both crutches to the hand on the affected side and reach back for the chair with the hand on the unaffected side
  —Lower yourself slowly into the chair

Warm and Cold Applications

Application of cold to a site slows blood flow to reduce pain, swelling, inflammation, and bleeding.

Procedure 14-5

Applying Cold Treatments

1. Assemble this equipment:
- Ice bag, ice collar, or disposable cold pack
- Cover
- Ice chips or small cubes
- Gauze or tape

2. Follow these Standard Precautions.

3. Fill the container about two-thirds full. Press it flat on a surface to express excess air from within. Seal the container.
Allows appliance to conform to patient contours; prevents leaks

4. If using a commercial pack, activate it now by following the package instructions.

5. Cover the bag.
Absorbs condensation; increases patient comfort

6. Greet and identify the patient. Explain the procedure.

7. Assess the area.
Provides baseline information for documentation; helps ensure that treatment can be successfully completed

8. Ensure the patient's comfort.
Promotes compliance

9. Secure the appliance with gauze or tape.
Provides greatest benefit; prevents pin punctures

10. Apply for no longer than 30 minutes.
Avoids rebound phenomenon

11. Assess the area for mottling, pallor, redness, or pain.
Allows reporting of adverse effects

12. If the treatment is to be reapplied, wait 1 hour.
Allows circulation to return to normal for tissue safety

13. Properly care for or dispose of equipment and supplies. Wash your hands.

14. Thank the patient and provide appropriate instructions.

Procedure Notes:

WARNING!

Commercial cold pack activators must be broken gently. They contain chemicals that can cause burns on contact. If a pack is leaking or is broken, dispose of it immediately.

14

You Need to Know:

- Check bags or collars for leaks to avoid wetting the patient.
- Small bits of ice conform to the patient's contours better than large pieces.
- Always cover appliances to increase patient comfort.
- Ice bags are used for larger areas; ice collars are used for smaller areas. Disposable cold packs are convenient and safe for most areas.
- Read the manufacturer's instructions for activating a commercial cold pack.
- Recommended temperature ranges are as follows: warm, 98°F to 115°F; cold, 95°F to 50°F.
- The young and the elderly respond to heat or cold differently than young adults. For those populations, use more conservative temperatures.
- If the patient reports adverse reactions to the therapy, instructions may need to be revised.

Applying a Warm or Cold Compress

Document on the Patient's Chart:
- Date and time
- Location of treatment
- Time of treatment
- Observations of treatment site
- Complications or patient complaints or concerns
- Patient education and instructions
- Your signature

EXAMPLE

7/16/2004	Cold pack applied to (L) lower leg.
1:00 PM	Pack removed at 1:30. No mottling,
	pallor, or redness noted. Pt. states
	pain is less. Pt. discharged to home
	with verbal and written instructions
	for cold application qid.
	—M. Sefferin, RMA

Instruct the Patient or Caregiver to:
- Report pain, tingling, erythema, or pallor during home therapy
- Cover the treatment method with an absorbable cloth covering, and remove the treatment after the prescribed time

Warm or cold compresses applied during appropriate healing stages help hasten the process.

Procedure 14-6

Applying a Warm or Cold Compress

1. Assemble this equipment:
   - Appropriate solution, warmed or cooled to the recommended temperature
   - Absorbent material of the physician's choice

- Waterproof barriers and insulators
- Thermometer
- Hot water bottle or ice pack (commercial hot or cold packs may be used)

2. Follow these Standard Precautions.

3. Pour the solution into the basin. Check the temperature of the solution.
Avoids injury to patient

4. Greet and identify the patient. Explain the procedure.

5. Ensure patient comfort and privacy.
Helps patient maintain position; protects privacy

6. Protect the undersurface and clothing with waterproof barriers.
Increases comfort

7. Put on gloves. Press or wring out excess moisture from the absorbent material. If using sterile procedure, this may be done with sterile gloves or with two sterile transfer forceps.
Avoids dripping on or overwetting patient

8. Touch the compress to the area lightly and observe the patient's reactions or ask for a response.
Reduces risk of pain or discomfort

9. Check the surface of the skin for reaction to the solution temperature.
Avoids inappropriate temperature

10. Gently arrange the compress over the area and conform the material to the patient's contours. Insulate the compress with waterproof barriers.
Ensures temperature transfer to patient; retards temperature loss

11. Check frequently for moisture and temperature. Hot water bottles or ice packs may be used to maintain the temperature.
Maintains fairly constant temperature

Applying a Warm or Cold Compress

Document on the Patient's Chart:
- Date and time
- Solution used
- Temperature of solution
- Location of treatment
- Time period of treatment
- Observations of the treatment site
- Complications or patient concerns or complaints
- Patient education and instructions
- Your signature

EXAMPLE

6/18/2004	Saline compresses at 110° applied
9:30 AM	to lesion on (R) forearm × 30 min.
	Skin warm and pink. Pt. given ver-
	bal and written instructions for
	applying compresses at home, ver-
	balized understanding.
	—S. Gomez, CMA

12. Discontinue after 30 minutes. Wait 1 hour before reapplying.

Avoids rebound phenomenon; allows circulation to return to normal for tissue safety

13. Discard disposable materials and appropriately disinfect reusable equipment. Wash your hands.

Procedure Notes:

WARNING!

Commercial pack activators (hot or cold) must be broken gently. They contain chemicals that can cause burns on contact. If a pack is leaking or is broken, dispose of it immediately.

Applying a Warm or Cold Compress

You Need to Know:

- If an open wound is present, observe surgical asepsis throughout the procedure.
- Review the procedures for asepsis and infection control for gloving procedures or for the use of transfer forceps if an open lesion is present and if sterile technique is required for this procedure.
- Warm compresses speed the suppuration process to hasten healing. Cold compresses slow bleeding and decrease inflammation.
- Because of the time involved, most compress treatments are performed by the patient or caregiver at home. You are likely to be responsible for patient or caregiver education (see Table 14-1 for additional guidelines).

Table 14-1

Proper Use of Heat and Cold: When Not to Use Heat or Cold—and Why

Do *not* use heat	Within 24 hours after an injury because it may increase bleeding
	For noninflammatory edema because increased capillary permeability allows additional tissue fluid to build up
	In cases of acute inflammation because increased blood supply increases the inflammatory process
	In the presence of malignancies because cell metabolism is enhanced
	Over the pregnant uterus because incidences of genetic mutation have been linked to heat applied to the gravid uterus
	On areas of erythema or vesicles because it compounds the existing problem
	Over metallic implants because it causes discomfort
Do *not* use cold	On open wounds because decreased blood supply delays healing
	In the presence of already-impaired circulation because it further impairs circulation

14

Using a Hot Water Bottle or Commercial Hot Pack

Here's how to provide heat to an area using a hot water bottle or commercial hot pack.

Procedure 14-7

Using a Hot Water Bottle or Commercial Hot Pack

1. Assemble this equipment:
   - Hot water bottle (with water at no more than 115°F) or commercial hot pack
   - Cover
   - Thermometer

2. Follow these Standard Precautions.

3. Fill bottle about two-thirds full with water at appropriate temperature. Check temperature with thermometer.
   Helps appliance conform to patient's contours; provides appropriate temperature

4. Place the bottle on a flat surface with the opening up and "burp" it by pressing out the excess air.
   Allows appliance to conform to patient's contours

5. If using a commercial hot pack, follow the manufacturer's directions for activating it.

6. Wrap and secure the pack or bottle before placing on the patient's skin.
   Increases comfort; helps prevent burns

7. Greet and identify the patient. Explain the procedure.

8. If continuous heat has been ordered, follow the physician's instructions; otherwise, remove after 30 minutes. Assess the area every 10 minutes.
   Avoids rebound phenomenon and allows circulation to return to normal

9. Report pallor (an indication of rebound), excessive redness (indicates that temperature may be too high for this lesion), or swelling (indicates that capillary permeability may contribute to tissue damage).
   Allows for evaluation of treatment plan

Document on the Patient's Chart:

- Date and time
- Location of treatment
- Time period of treatment
- Observations of the treatment site
- Complications or patient complaints or concerns
- Patient education and instructions
- Your signature

EXAMPLE

12/16/2004	Pt. given verbal and written in-
3:00 PM	structions on application of hot
	water bottle for use at home qid
	× 30 min to muscle pain, (L)
	thigh. Verbalized understanding.
	—R. Smith, CMA

14

10. Caution the patient that the body adapts to the temperature and that it is not necessary to continually increase the temperature to achieve maximum benefits.
Protects patient from injury

Procedure Notes:

WARNING!

Commercial pack activators must be broken gently. They contain chemicals that can cause burns on contact. If a pack is leaking or is broken, dispose of it immediately.

Assisting With Therapeutic Soaks

- See guidelines in Procedure 14-5 for temperature ranges.
- Because of the time involved, most hot water bottle or commercial hot pack treatments are performed by the patient or caregiver at home. You are likely to be responsible for patient or caregiver education.

How should you soak a large area of the body?

Procedure 14-8

Assisting With Therapeutic Soaks

1. Assemble this equipment:
- Container large enough to comfortably contain the part to be soaked
- Solution (at no more than 110°F)
- Towels (for padding surfaces and drying the part)
- Thermometer

2. Follow these Standard Precautions.

3. Fill the container with the solution and check the temperature with the thermometer. The proper temperature is usually no more than 110°F because of the large surface involved and the possibility of blood pressure changes with vasodilation.
Prevents burns or other tissue damage

4. Greet and identify the patient. Explain the procedure.

5. Slowly lower the part into the container and check for the patient's reaction. Arrange the part comfortably and in easy alignment. Check for pressure areas and pad the edges. The bottom may also be padded for comfort.
Allows patient to adjust to temperature

6. Soak for the prescribed period of time.
Prevents tissue damage or rebound phenomenon

7. Check every 5 to 10 minutes for the proper temperature. If additional water or solution must be added to maintain the temperature, remove a quantity of the solution. With your hand between the patient and the stream of solution, add the required amount and swirl it quickly through the container.
Maintains maximum benefit; avoids patient discomfort from solution

8. Soak for the prescribed time, usually 15 to 20 minutes.
Prevents tissue damage or rebound

9. Carefully dry the part.
Prevents discomfort from chilling or brisk rubbing of sensitive skin

10. Assess the area.

11. Thank the patient and provide appropriate instructions.

12. Properly care for or dispose of equipment supplies. Wash your hands.

Procedure Notes:

14

You Need to Know:

• See guidelines in Procedure 14-5 for temperature ranges.
• Because of the time involved, therapeutic soaks are usually performed by the patient or caregiver at home. You are likely to be responsible for patient or caregiver education.

Instruct the Patient or Caregiver Regarding:

• Performance of soaks at home: a large foam cooler works well to maintain the proper temperature, to allow the extremity to rest comfortably, and to be completely submerged; a towel placed over the opening helps maintain the optimum temperature.

Document on the Patient's Chart:

- Date and time
- Location of treatment
- Time period of treatment
- Type of solution
- Observations of the treatment site
- Complications or patient complaints or concerns
- Patient education and instructions
- Your signature

EXAMPLE

5/8/2004	(L) foot soaked × 20 min in warm
10:45 AM	water (110°) as ordered. Skin warm
	and pink after soaking, states
	muscle and joint pain slightly
	relieved.
	—E. West, RMA

14

General Procedures

Should the injured arm be supported while the patient moves about? A sling helps relieve pressure and keeps the hand in position.

Procedure 14-9

Applying a Triangular Arm Sling

1. Assemble this equipment:
   - Sling as ordered by the physician
   - Pins
2. Follow these Standard Precautions.

3. Greet and identify the patient. Explain the procedure and ask for questions.

4. Position the affected limb with the hand at slightly less than a 90° angle so that the fingers are higher than the elbow.
Reduces swelling

5. Place the triangle with the uppermost corner at the shoulder on the unaffected side (extend the corner across the nape); the middle angle at the elbow of the affected side; and the final, lowermost corner pointing toward the foot on the unaffected side.
Allows proper positioning

6. Bring up the lowermost corner to meet the upper corner at the side of the neck, never at the back of the neck.
Avoids pressure from the knot against the neck

7. Tie or pin the sling. Secure the elbow by fitting any extra fabric neatly around the limb and pinning it. (Figure 14-2 shows appropriate sling application.)
Secures sling

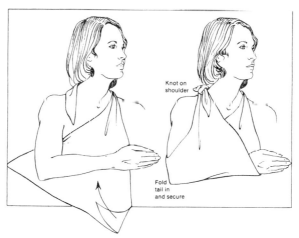

Figure 14-2. Triangular arm sling application.

Document on the Patient's Chart:

- Date and time
- Limb involved
- Observations of patient reaction
- Application of appliance
- Patient complaints or concerns
- Patient education and instructions
- Your signature

EXAMPLE

1/14/2004	Short arm cast applied to (L) arm
11:15 AM	per Dr. Watson. Arm sling applied,
	pt. instructed on cast care and
	sling application at home. (L) fingers
	warm and pink with good movement
	—J. Carr, CMA

14

8. Check the patient's comfort level and distal extremity circulation.

Ensures compliance and patient safety

Procedure Notes:

You Need to Know:

- Fitted canvas slings with Velcro or buckles are also available and are becoming the appliances of choice.

Instruct the Patient or Caregiver to:

- Call with concerns or questions
- Keep the hand elevated to avoid swelling
- Tie the knot away from the back of the neck

How can you make colon procedures more effective and less disturbing to your patient?

Procedure 14-10

Preparing the Patient for Colon Procedures

1. Assemble this equipment:
   - Appropriate instrument (flexible or rigid sigmoido-scope, anoscope, or proctoscope)
   - Water-soluble lubricant
   - Fenestrated drape or gown
   - Cotton swabs
   - Suction source (if not part of the scope)
   - Biopsy forceps
   - Specimen container with preservative
   - Completed laboratory requests
   - Personal wipes
   - Equipment for assessing vital signs

2. Follow these Standard Precautions.

14

3. Check the illumination of the light source. Turn off the power to avoid a buildup of heat.
   Ensures that all equipment is functional

4. Greet and identify the patient. Explain the procedure.

5. Instruct the patient to empty bladder.
   Decreases discomfort

6. Assess and record the vital signs.
   Provides baseline for monitoring

7. Have the patient undress from the waist down or undress completely and put on a gown opening in the back.

8. Assist the patient onto the table. If the instrument of choice is an anoscope or fiberoptic device, Sims position or a left-lying position is most comfortable for the patient. If a rigid instrument is used, the patient may as-

sume a knee-chest position or be placed on a proctologic table that supports the patient in a knee-chest position.
Repositions abdominal contents into abdominal cavity rather than pelvis to facilitate procedure

9. When the patient is in position, drape properly. A fenestrated drape is usually used.

10. Continually monitor the patient's response and offer reassurance during the examination. Instruct the patient to breathe slowly through pursed lips to aid in relaxation.

11. Assist the physician as needed with lubricants, instruments, power sources, swabs, biopsy equipment, and specimen containers.

12. After the procedure, assist the patient into a comfortable position and allow a rest period. Offer personal cleaning wipes and assist with cleaning as needed. Monitor the vital signs before allowing the patient to stand. Assist the patient from the table, and remain close at hand to prevent falls.
Promotes comfort and safety

13. Have the patient dress. Help as needed.

14. Thank the patient and give appropriate instructions.

15. Clean the room. Route the specimens to the proper laboratory. Clean or dispose of the supplies and equipment as appropriate, and wash your hands.

Procedure Notes:

14

You Need to Know:

- Do not ask the patient to assume the knee-chest position until the physician is ready to begin. This position is difficult to maintain, and the patient may become faint.
- Instructions should have been given to the patient several days before the procedure regarding colon cleansing (see Box 14-2). If the preparatory protocol was not followed, the procedure should be explained again and rescheduled.
- Some patients are ordered a mild sedative before the procedure.

BOX 14-2

Patient Preparation for Bowel Studies

Many bowel studies, such as barium enema and flexible sigmoidoscopy, require that the bowel be completely clear of fecal matter for the test to be considered diagnostic. With minor variations as directed by the physician, the bowel preparation will include the following:

- Liquid diet without dairy products for the full day before the procedure or a clear liquid evening meal
- A laxative the evening preceding the procedure; enemas also may be ordered
- NPO except water after midnight through the time of the procedure
- Rectal suppository, Fleet enema, or cleansing enema the morning of the procedure

If inflammatory processes or ulcerations are suspected, only gentle cleansing will be used to avoid undue discomfort or possible perforation of lesions.

14

WARNING!

Colon examination procedures may cause cardiac arrhythmias and a change in blood pressure in some patients. Carefully monitor the patient's response during the procedure and alert the physician if the patient seems distressed.

Instruct the Patient Regarding:

- Pressure and the urge to defecate during the procedure; this eases as the procedure progresses
- Gas pressure when air is insufflated; this also eases

Document on the Patient's Chart:

- Date and time
- Colon preparation and adherence to protocol
- Patient complaints or concerns
- Patient education and instructions
- Your signature

EXAMPLE

5/31/2004	CC: colonoscopy scheduled for to-
12:45 PM	day, pt. states he followed bowel
	prep as ordered. T 98 (0), P 76,
	R 16, BP 120/80 (R).
	—S. Clay, CMA

An object in the eye? Use extreme caution to prevent further injury.

14

Procedure 14-11

Removing a Foreign Object From the Eye

1. Assemble this equipment:
   - Sterile, cotton-tipped applicator
   - Sterile water or saline
   - Sterile medicine dropper or small bulb syringe
   - Tissues
   - Sterile gauze

2. Follow these Standard Precautions.

3. Greet and identify the patient. Explain the procedure.

4. Glove now. With the gauze against the cheek, pull down the lower eyelid and check for the object. If it is seen,

moisten the applicator with the water or saline and gently try to remove the object.

Avoids potential exposure to body fluids

5. If the object is not found on the lower lid, grasp the lashes of the upper lid and pull gently upward, checking the upper surfaces of the eye for the object.

6. Perform an eye irrigation if necessary, following the steps in Procedure 11-9: Irrigating the Eye.

7. Wipe away any liquid with the tissue. Remove and dispose of gloves.

8. Properly care for or dispose of equipment and supplies. Clean the work area. Wash your hands.

Procedure Notes:

You Need to Know:

- Embedded objects must be removed by a physician, but loose debris may be removed by the medical assistant.
- Question the patient about his tetanus immunization if the foreign body pierced the mucous membrane of the eye.

14

Instruct the Patient to:

- Prevent eye injuries by wearing protective eyewear during procedures that may result in injuries by foreign bodies

Document on the Patient's Chart:
- Date and time
- Removal of the foreign body
- Description of the foreign body, including size
- Patient complaints or concerns
- Results of any eye tests performed to determine extent of damage, as needed
- Full documentation of irrigation, if performed
- Full documentation of medication, if administered
- Notification of physician
- Patient education and instructions
- Your signature

EXAMPLE

5/5/2004	CC: c/o metal chip in his OD—
9:35 AM	accident occurred on the job × 30
	min ago. Foreign object removed
	from OD per Dr. Spruce. Neosporin
	ophthalmic ointment instilled in
	OD, patch applied. To RTO tomor-
	row for recheck.
	—J. Smith, RMA

14

LABORATORY PROCEDURES

15

Opening and Closing the Physician's Office Laboratory

How should you begin your day in the physician's office laboratory (POL)?

Procedure 15-1

Opening the Physician's Office Laboratory

1. Wash your hands on entering the laboratory.

2. Review the checklist of the day's scheduled activities.

3. Unlock doors as appropriate and turn on lights as needed; turn off disinfecting ultraviolet lights if in use.

4. Turn on all equipment or change mode from standby to ready to allow it to warm up.

5. Check and record temperature readings on all incubators, refrigerators, freezers, and water baths.

6. Remove from refrigerator all kits and reagents that must be at room temperature for testing.

7. Put on PPE gown as needed to perform procedures.

8. Run all appropriate daily controls as required for quality assurance/quality control program.

9. Perform any necessary equipment repair, cleaning, or maintenance before use. (This may be done the previous evening.)

10. Prepare fresh 10% bleach solution and fill dispensing bottles, or check that disinfectant solutions to be used have not expired.

11. Disinfect all working areas with 10% bleach or other appropriate solutions.

12. Check laboratory inventory and properly dispose of all expired or damaged materials and reagents.

13. Restock necessary laboratory supplies, noting items that should be ordered.

14. Autoclave, disinfect, or sanitize equipment and supplies as needed.

15. Sign off daily activities on checklist as completed.

16. Retrieve a list of specialty tests scheduled for the day, and make sure all necessary supplies and equipment are ready and available for use.

17. Retrieve any uncharted or unreported test results from the previous workday; circle abnormal values and attach the reports to the patients' charts. Report to the physician and record all test results in patients' charts.

18. Ensure that weekly and occasional activities assigned to the day are addressed. Initial all items on checklist.

Procedure Notes:

You Need to Know:

- This list may vary depending on the type of office, its location, and the physician's needs.

What should you do before leaving the POL for the day?

Procedure 15-2

Closing the Physician's Office Laboratory

1. Prepare the checklist for the next day's scheduled activities.

2. Make sure all specimens are processed, tested, routed for testing, or stored away for the next day.

3. Check that all pending procedures have been performed. Check with the physician and clinical assistant before securing the laboratory equipment.

4. Store all kits, reagents, plates, and supplies. Check that all supplies are labeled with the date that they were received, the date they were opened, and the initials of the worker who prepared them.

5. Clean the work area and dispose of waste properly.

6. Autoclave, disinfect, or sanitize any equipment or supplies as appropriate.

7. Disinfect all work areas.

8. Bag all biohazard waste if appropriate and dispose of properly.

9. Turn off all equipment, or switch mode to standby if appropriate.

10. Restock any necessary laboratory supply items.

11. Wash your hands before leaving the laboratory. Lock doors as necessary and turn off the lights as appropriate. Turn on disinfecting ultraviolet lights.

15

Procedure Notes:

You Need to Know:

• This list may vary depending on the type of office, its location, and the physician's needs.

Specimen Collection and Testing

Pathogens in the respiratory system may be identified using this method.

Procedure 16-1

Collecting a Specimen for a Throat Culture

1. Assemble this equipment:
   - Tongue blade or depressor
   - Sterile specimen container
   - Sterile swab if one is not supplied with the specimen container
   - Completed laboratory request slip

2. Follow these Standard Precautions.

3. Greet and identify the patient. Explain the procedure.

4. Have the patient sit with a light source directed at the throat.
   Assists with visualization of areas of concern

5. Put on gloves and face mask or shield.

6. Carefully remove the sterile swab from the container.
   Ensures sterility

7. Have the patient say "ahhh" as you press on the mid-point of the tongue with the tongue depressor.
   Raises uvula and decreases gag urge

8. Swab the areas of concern on the mucous membranes, especially the tonsillar area, the crypts, and the posterior pharynx. Turn the swab to expose all of its surfaces. Avoid touching areas other than those suspected of infections.
Ensures maximum specimen collection

9. Maintain the tongue depressor position while withdrawing the swab.
Avoids contaminating the swab with saliva

10. Follow the instructions on the specimen container for transferring the swab. Some require that the wooden swab be broken after being dropped into the culture; others may have a special swab that is contained within the cap and is secured when the container is sealed.
Ensures specimen integrity

11. Label the specimen with the patient's name; the date; the identification number; and the specific location from which the specimen was taken, for example, right tonsillar area or posterior oropharynx.
Provides proper identification

12. Thank the patient and give appropriate instructions.

13. Properly dispose of the equipment and supplies. Remove gloves and wash your hands.

14. Route the specimen or store it appropriately until routing can be completed.
Maintains specimen integrity

16

Procedure Notes:

You Need to Know:

- If you place the tongue depressor too far forward, it will not be effective. If you place it too far back, it will gag the patient unnecessarily.

Document on the Patient's Chart:

- Date and time
- Collection of throat culture
- Routing of specimen
- Patient complaints and concerns
- Patient education and instructions
- Your signature

EXAMPLE

11/05/04	Pt. arrived in office complaining of
0937	sore throat × 2 days. Febrile:
	103°. Throat culture ordered by Dr.
	Andrews. Throat specimen ob-
	tained from posterior pharynx and
	bilateral pharyngeal arches.
	Routed to lab. To call in AM for re-
	sults and treatment options.
	—C. Davis, CMA

16

Many gastrointestinal disorders can be diagnosed by a properly collected and processed stool specimen.

Procedure 16-2

Collecting a Stool Specimen

1. Assemble this equipment:
   - Stool specimen container (usually waxed cardboard or plastic to avoid the transfer of pathogens through a moist container)
   - Wooden spatulas or tongue blades

- Bedpan with cover or toilet collection container (popularly called a "nun's cap" or "Mexican hat") with cover
- Personal wipes for the patient

2. Follow these Standard Precautions.

3. Greet and identify the patient. Explain the procedure.

4. Tell the patient to defecate in the bedpan or toilet collection container, not the toilet. The patient must void urine separately. Make sure the patient discards toilet tissue in the toilet and not in the bedpan or collection container.
   Avoids contaminating specimen with water, urine, or toilet tissue

5. Put on gloves and obtain the bedpan or collection container from the patient.
   Reduces exposure to pathogens

6. Using a tongue blade or wooden spatula, remove small portions of the stool from the bedpan or collection container. Take the specimens from the first and final portions of the stool.
   Provides the most concentrated substances required for testing

7 Transfer the stool to the specimen container. Do not allow feces to soil the outer surface of the specimen container.

8. Discard the supplies in biohazard containers, and flush the remaining stool.

9. Cap the specimen quickly and tightly.
   Prevents moisture loss, which may alter results

10. Assist the patient with cleaning the rectal area. Have the patient wash his hands.
    Provides comfort; prevents spread of pathogens

11. Thank the patient and provide appropriate instructions.

16

12. Clean, disinfect, and store or properly dispose of the bedpan or collection container. Remove gloves and wash hands after handling the specimen and supplies.

13. Label the specimen and attach the laboratory requests.
Provides proper identification

14. Store the specimen as directed.
Maintains specimen integrity

Procedure Notes:

You Need to Know:

- Some stool specimens require refrigeration, others are kept at room temperature, and some must be incubated. Check the office policy and procedure manual for recommendations for storage and routing of all specimens.
- If blood is present in the stool, be sure to include samples in the specimen, because greater concentrations of pathogens may be present in these areas.
- Most patients are instructed to bring in the morning stool rather than giving a specimen in the office. You may be required to relay proper instructions and provide the patient with education brochures and supplies.

16

Instruct the Patient or Caregiver to:

- Collect from the first and final portions of the stool for greater concentrations of substances of concern
- Include samples of specimens containing blood for possible greater concentrations of substances of concern
- Avoid urinating into the specimen container or including toilet tissue; either may contaminate the specimen

Document on the Patient's Chart:

- Date and time
- Collection of specimen and time received (if it is to be routed)
- Description of specimen as needed
- Routing of specimen
- Occult blood test results if performed before routing specimen
- Your signature

	(Note: See Procedure 16-1 for
	charting example.)

Small amounts of blood are not always visible in the stool. This test screens for gastrointestinal bleeding.

Procedure 16-3

Testing for Occult Blood

1. Assemble this equipment:
   - Patient's labeled specimen pack
   - Developers or reagents

2. Follow these Standard Precautions.

3. Identify the patient's pack, or receive the specimen from the physician.
   Proper identification prevents errors; prompt testing helps ensure accuracy.

4. Open the test window on the back of the pack and apply the testing reagent or developer. Read the color change at the specified time, usually 60 seconds. Apply devel-

16

Document on the Patient's Chart:

- Date and time
- Testing results
- Notification of physician
- Patient complaints or concerns
- Patient education and instructions
- Your signature

EXAMPLE

6/13/04	Pt. was instructed on previous
1500	visit (6-11-04) to collect a stool
	specimen on Hemoccult Test Pak.
	Pt. returned today with kit.
	Pt. states he followed directions.
	Test results positive. Dr. Franklyn
	alerted to the findings.
	—A. Jones, CMA

16

opers as directed onto the control monitor section of the pack. Wait the specified time.
Ensures accurate results

5. Properly dispose of the pack, gloves, and supplies. Wash your hands.

Procedure Notes:

You Need to Know:

- Depending on the method of testing, the specimen may be tested as quickly as 3 to 5 minutes after collection or up to 14 days if properly stored.

- Check with the patient before testing the specimen to ensure that dietary restrictions were followed; if they were not, the test result is invalid.

Instruct the Patient or Caregiver Regarding:

- Test directions
- Importance of following dietary restrictions exactly as specified to avoid having to repeat the test

How can you help identify respiratory illnesses from deep within the lungs?

Procedure 16-4

Collecting a Sputum Specimen

1. Assemble this equipment:
   - Labeled sterile specimen container
   - Cover bag

2. Follow these Standard Precautions.

3. Greet and identify the patient. Explain the procedure.

4. Have the patient brush her teeth or rinse her mouth well.
   Avoids contaminating specimen with food particles

5. Put on gloves and face shield and impervious gown, if you are assisting with collection.

6. Have the patient cough deeply, using the abdominal muscles as well as the accessory muscles to bring up secretions from the lung fields and not just the upper airways.
   Ensures that the specimen contains pathogens from lungs and not throat

7. Have the patient expectorate directly into the specimen container without touching the inside and without getting sputum on the sides of the container. About 5 to 10 mL is usually needed.
   Prevents contaminating outside of container

16

8. Handle the specimen observing Standard Precautions (see step 2). Cap the container immediately and drop it into the cover container.

   Avoids exposure to potentially hazardous material

9. Label the specimen with the patient's name, the date, and the identification number.

   Provides identification of specimen

10. Assist the patient to rinse her mouth after collecting the specimen.

    Promotes patient comfort

11. Thank the patient and give appropriate instructions.

12. Properly care for or dispose of equipment and supplies. Clean the work area. Remove gloves, gown, and face shield, and wash your hands.

13. Process the specimen immediately, or within 2 hours, to avoid compromising the study results.

    Allows for accuracy in testing

Procedure Notes:

16

WARNING!

Be aware that any sputum on the outside of the specimen container is potentially hazardous.

You Need to Know:

- Proper handling of the specimen is essential to ensure an accurate result. Improper handling may result in proliferation, overgrowth, or death of the pathogen, causing a false result.

Instruct the Patient to:

- Cough deeply to ensure that the specimen is mucus from the lungs, not saliva from the mouth
- Practice good oral hygiene
- Cover the mouth and nose when coughing to avoid transmitting pathogens to family members and caregivers

Document on the Patient's Chart:

- Date and time
- Performance of the procedure
- Routing of specimen
- Patient complaints or concerns
- Patient education and instructions
- Your signature

11/03/04	S: "I have an awful cough."
1030	O: 80-year-old COPD pt. Complain-
	ing of dyspnea × 3 days and a
	productive cough. Sputum green-
	ish-yellow in color. Crackles in left
	lower lung field. T: 102°.
	A: Productive cough
	P: 1. Sputum collected per order of
	Dr. Raymond. Pt. instructed
	in collection procedure. Ap-
	proximately 10 mL of dark yel-
	low, thick mucus obtained.
	2. Specimen routed to CGH lab.

continued

16

	3. Pt. educated about need to
	stop smoking. Hygiene instruc-
	tions given on covering nose
	and mouth when coughing. Pt.
	verbalized understanding of all
	instructions and pt. education
	brochure.
	4. Dr. Raymond ordered CXR. Pt.
	given directions to Radiology
	Dept. at CGH.
	—Jackie Shapiro, CMA

16

17

Clinical Chemistry

Does your patient need blood glucose monitoring? The Accu-Chek Compact is one method of assessment.

Note: There are many types of blood glucose monitors. Be sure to follow specific manufacturer's instructions.

Procedure 17-1

Determining Blood Glucose Using the Accu-Check Compact

1. Assemble this equipment:
   - Accu-Check Compact analyzer
   - Glucose strip test drum
   - Lancet
   - Alcohol pad
   - Sterile gauze
   - Paper towel

2. Follow these Standard Precautions.

3. Identify the patient and wash your hands.
   Proper patient identification is critical; handwashing lets the patient know you are thorough in your technique.

4. Install the test drum.

   a. With the meter off, slide the release button toward the display to open the drum compartment.

   b. If there is a used drum in the compartment, hold the meter upright to remove the used drum.
     Allows the old test drum to simply drop out

   c. Remove the new test drum from its vial.

   d. Slide the new drum onto the plastic post inside the compartment. It can only be inserted in one direction.

   e. Close the compartment door until it snaps.
     Note:
- Once you remove a test drum from its vial, you have 90 days to use up all of the strips.
- Do not open the drum compartment until you have used all the strips. Doing so makes the 90-day use-by date invalid.
- If you take out a partially used test drum and put it back in the meter, "CTRL" flashes in the display, meaning you should perform a control test.
- Keep the test drum vial or vial label until you are finished with the test drum. You will need to refer to the numbers on the label when you run control tests.
- When the drum is empty, a dot appears in the view window on the back of the meter and "End" and the test drum symbol flash on the display.
- Store the drum and meter in a cool dry place. DO NOT put them in the refrigerator.
- Be sure all controls are satisfactorily completed before patient testing.

5. Open the display cover and press the test button.
Turns the analyzer and ejects a strip for testing

6. When you see the test strip at the bottom of the meter and the flashing hand and blood drop, set the meter down and perform the capillary puncture.
Automatically sets the analyzer for testing, and you have 5 minutes after the strip appears to perform the test

17

7. Once the puncture is complete, immediately touch and hold the blood drop to the black notch on the front edge of the strip. The blood is drawn into the test strip automatically.

   Do not pull the finger away until the meter beeps or the 000 is displayed; you may apply more blood for up to 25 seconds after applying the first drop.

8. The 000 on the display gradually disappears, and the test result is displayed.

   Test results will automatically be stored in the meter's memory.

9. Holding the meter upright, press the test button to release the test strip and turn the meter off.

10. Wash your hands.

11. Dispose of all used materials in the proper waste receptacles.

12. Record the results in the chart.

Procedure Notes:

WARNING!

If the glucose level is higher or lower than expected, refer to the troubleshooting guide provided by the manufacturer.

17

You Need to Know:

- Quality assurance measure. Controls are available in the low, normal, and high range to ensure that the glucose meter is functioning properly. These controls should be tested daily or as recommended by the manufacturer (per test drum) or every time a patient glucose test is performed if the meter is not used daily.

Instruct the Patient to:

- Avoid eating, drinking, smoking, or chewing gum for at least 8 hours before test time if a fasting test is scheduled
- Test glucose levels regularly and document results to evaluate the efficiency of treatment

Glucose Tolerance Testing (GTT)

Document on the Patient's Chart:
- Date and time
- Testing site
- Test results
- Action taken (if any)
- Patient education
- Your signature

EXAMPLE

3/5/04	Lancet skin puncture right index
3:00 PM	finger. Glucose tested with Accu-
	Check Compact. Results: 60
	mg/dL. Dr. Peters was notified. Pt.
	was given a glass of orange juice.
	—Mysti Rogers, CMA

- Obtain a blood sample using the proper technique (provide instructions, if necessary)
- Avoid self-regulating insulin therapy, which can be dangerous
- Recognize the signs and symptoms of high or low glucose levels, and know the treatments for each

17

How does your patient metabolize his glucose intake? This test provides an extended overview.

Procedure 17-2

Glucose Tolerance Testing (GTT)

1. Assemble this equipment:
   - Calibrated amount of glucose per the physician's order
   - Phlebotomy equipment
   - Glucose test strips
   - Glucose meter equipment

- Alcohol wipes
- Stopwatch

2. Follow these Standard Precautions.

3. Obtain a fasting blood sugar (FBS) specimen (red top) from the patient, using the steps outlined in the venipuncture procedure (Procedure 20-1). Test the specimen glucose level.

   Note: If the glucose level is over 140 mg/dL, do not proceed with the test. Notify the physician that the patient's fasting glucose level is over 140 mg/dL and get new orders. If it is less than 140, you may proceed with the test.

   Provides baseline for further interpretation

4. Administer the glucose drink to the patient, to be consumed within a 5-minute period. Note the time the patient finishes the drink; this is the start time of the test.

   Ensures appropriate evaluation of glucose metabolism

5. Exactly 30 minutes after the patient has finished the glucose drink, obtain another blood specimen by venipuncture.

   Provides for precise timing of specimen collection for accurate interpretation of results

6. Exactly 1 hour after the glucose drink, repeat step 5.

7. Exactly 2 hours after the glucose drink, repeat step 5.

8. Exactly 3 hours after the glucose drink, repeat step 5. Unless a GTT of longer than 3 hours has been requested, the testing is complete at this time. (For a longer GTT, continue specimen collection in the same manner for as many additional hours as required.)

9. If the specimens are to be tested by an outside laboratory, package as required and arrange for transportation.

   Helps ensure quality samples

10. Properly care for or dispose of equipment and supplies. Clean the work area. Wash your hands.

17

Glucose Tolerance Testing (GTT)

Procedure Notes:

WARNING!

· It is recommended that laboratories test the blood sample before you administer the glucose drink; if the FBS exceeds a certain reading (e.g., greater than 140 mg/dL), do not perform the GTT. Notify the physician.

· If the patient experiences any severe symptoms (e.g., headache, dizziness, vomiting), end the test and notify the physician. These symptoms could be the result of glucose levels that are too high or too low for the patient to tolerate.

You Need to Know:

• Ensure that the patient remains fairly sedentary throughout this procedure (e.g., no long walks between blood draws); exercising alters the glucose level by burning glucose for more energy. The patient should avoid smoking because it may artificially increase the glucose level. Only water should be ingested.

• Label each specimen with the patient's name and time of collection.

Instruct the Patient or Caregiver to:

• Test glucose levels regularly and document results to evaluate the efficiency of treatment

• Obtain a blood sample using the proper technique (provide instructions, if necessary)

• Avoid self-regulating insulin therapy, which can be dangerous

• Recognize the signs and symptoms of high or low glucose levels, and know the treatments for each

17

Document on the Patient's Chart:
- Date and time
- Test results, if performed on site
- Patient observations
- Patient education
- Your signature

9/15/04	GTT test:
0800	0800 FBS: 100 mg/dL glucose
	0810 Glucose drink given to pt.
	0815 Glucose drink finished
	0845 Glucose: 125 mg/dL
	0915 Glucose: 132 mg/dL
	1015 Glucose: 120 mg/dL
	1115 Glucose: 110 mg/dL
	Pt. tolerated procedure well, dis-
	charged by Dr. Lynoh.
	—S. Collins, RMA

17

Hematology

How do you determine the number and types of white blood cells in a patient sample?

Procedure 18-1

Performing a Manual WBC Count

1. Assemble this equipment:
   - Unopette system for white blood cell (WBC) count
   - Neubauer hemacytometer
   - Coverslip
   - Gauze
   - Moist filter paper or moist cotton ball
   - Petri dish
   - Hand tally counter

2. Follow these Standard Precautions.

3. Using the shield on the capillary pipette, pierce the diaphragm in the neck of the reservoir, pushing the tip of the shield firmly through the diaphragm before removing it. Remove the shield from the capillary pipette using a twisting motion. Fill the pipette with free-flowing whole blood obtained through skin puncture, or from a properly obtained, well-mixed EDTA (purple-topped tube) specimen.

4. If filling from a tube, place the tip of the Unopette just below the surface of the blood. Allow capillary action to fill the Unopette system completely.

5. Wipe off the pipette with gauze, being careful not to draw gauze across the tip.
   Prevents erroneous results if gauze touches and absorbs some of the blood sample; removes surface contaminants

6. Squeeze the reservoir gently to press the air out without expelling any of the specimen. Place your index finger over the opening of the overflow chamber of the pipette.
   Prevents loss of blood from the assembly

7. Maintain the pressure on the reservoir and your finger position on the pipette and insert the pipette into the reservoir.
   Allows an entry for the specimen into the reservoir

8. Release the reservoir pressure, then remove your finger from the pipette.
   Allows the specimen to enter the reservoir

9. Gently press and release the reservoir several times, forcing the diluent into but not out of the overflow chamber.
   Ensures an accurate dilution without destroying fragile cells

10. Place your index finger over the opening of the overflow chamber and gently invert or swirl the container several times. Remove your finger and cover the opening with the pipette shield.
    Maintains integrity of the specimen while mixing with diluent; prevents leakage and evaporation

11. Label with the required patient information and set the unit aside for 10 minutes.
    Ensures proper patient identification; allows the red blood cells to lyse

12. At the proper interval, mix the contents again by gently swirling the assembly.

13. Remove the pipette from the Unopette reservoir and replace it as a dropper assembly.
    Allows the diluted specimen to charge the hemacytometer

18

14. Invert the reservoir and gently squeeze the sides, discarding the first three to four drops.
Cleans the capillary lumen of specimen that might not be adequately mixed

15. Charge the hemacytometer by touching the tip of the assembly to the V-shaped loading area of the covered chamber. Control the flow gently and do not overfill. Do not allow the specimen to flow into the H-shaped moats that surround the platform loading area.
Prevents overfilling and forming bubbles

16. Place the hemacytometer and the moistened filter paper or cotton ball in the Petri dish and cover the entire assembly for 5 to 10 minutes.
Prevents drying, allows the cells to settle

17. Place the prepared hemacytometer on the microscope stage and turn to the 100× magnification (Figure 18-1).
Prepares for the cell count

18. Using a zigzag counting pattern, starting at the top far left, count the top row left to right. At the end of the top row, drop to the second row and count from right to left.
Avoids omitting cells

18

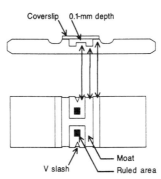

Figure 18-1. The Neubauer hemacytometer.

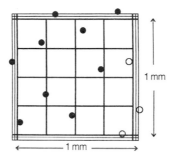

Figure 18-2. Rules for microscopic counting of leukocytes on the Neubauer hemacytometer. One square millimeter is illustrated. Leukocytes are counted in nine of these 1-mm squares. Leukocytes that touch the top or left triple boundary lines are counted; those that touch the bottom or right boundaries are not. (Solid circle, cells counted; open circle, cells not counted.)

19. Using the tally counter, count all of the WBCs within the boundaries and those that touch the top and left borders. Do not count those that touch the bottom or right borders (Figure 18-2).

Prevents inaccurate estimation of cells

Procedure Notes:

You Need to Know:

18

- Automated cell counters are used in almost all physicians' office laboratories to eliminate the subjectivity of manual cell counts.

Document on the Patient's Chart:

- Date and time
- Performance of procedure
- Site of venipuncture
- Results of testing
- Action taken, if any
- Patient education and instructions
- Your signature

5/15/04	Venipuncture to left antecubitus.
2:00 PM	Hematology results as follows:
	WBC: 4,880
	WBC diff:
	Neutrophils 60%
	Lymphocytes 25%
	Monocytes 5%
	Eosinophils 8%
	Basophils 2%
	RBC: 4.6
	Hgb 17 mg/dL
	Hct 50%
	MCV 88
	Platelets 250,000
	ESR 16
	PT 18
	PTT 45
	—Erik Williams, RMA

18

Prepare a specimen for evaluation of blood cells in this manner.

Procedure 18-2

Performing a Manual RBC Count

1. Assemble this equipment:
   - Unopette system for red blood cell (RBC) count
   - Clean, lint-free hemacytometer
   - Coverslip
   - Gauze
   - Moist filter paper or moist cotton ball
   - Petri dish
   - Microscope
   - Hand tally counter

2. Follow these Standard Precautions.

3. **to 16.** Follow the steps listed in Procedure 18-1: Performing a Manual WBC Count.

17. Place the hemacytometer on the microscope stage so that the ruled area can be surveyed with the low-power objective. Focus the microscope, then progress to the 40× magnification to count the RBCs.
    Ensures proper positioning and magnification for counting

18. Count the RBCs in the four corner squares and the center square, following the zigzag pattern described in Procedure 18-1. Starting at the top far left, count the top row left to right. At the end of the top row, drop to the second row and count from right to left. Continue this pattern until all of the rows are counted. Count cells touching the upper and left side, but do not count those on the lower and right side.
    Eliminates confusion and overcounting or undercounting

19. Tally the count and record the number. Return the counter to 0 and count the next grid. Count the opposite side of the hemacytometer.

18

20. The count within the squares should not vary by more than 20 cells. If the variable is greater, the test must be repeated.
Ensures accuracy of testing

21. Average the two sides and multiply to result by 10,000.
Gives the total number of RBCs per mm3

22. Clean the hemacytometer and coverslip with 10% bleach and wipe dry with lens paper. Dispose of or care for any other equipment and supplies appropriately. Clean the work area. Remove gloves and gown and wash your hands.
Ensures that equipment/supplies are available for next use; prevents spread of microorganisms

Procedure Notes:

WARNING!

Be very careful when washing coverslip. It is a specific weight for the hematocytometer and can be easily cracked or broken.

You Need to Know:

- Automated cell counters are used in almost all physicians' office laboratories to eliminate the subjectivity of manual cell counts. (Note: See Procedure 18-1 for documentation guidelines and charting example.)

18

Does the physician need to know if a patient is anemic?

Procedure 18-3

Making a Peripheral Blood Smear

1. Assemble this equipment:
- Clean glass slides with frosted ends
- Pencil
- Transfer pipette
- Whole blood

- Appropriate biohazard barrier devices
- Well-mixed patient specimen

2. Follow these Standard Precautions.

3. Obtain an EDTA (purple-topped tube) blood specimen from the patient using the proper venipuncture technique (Procedure 20-1).

4. Label the slide on the frosted area.
Ensures that markings are retained during staining

5. Place a drop of blood 1 cm from the frosted end of the slide.

6. Place the slide on a flat surface; with the thumb and forefinger of the right hand hold the second (spreader) slide against the surface of the first at a 30° angle, and draw it back against the drop of blood until contact is established (Figure 18-3). Allow the blood to spread out under the edge, and then push the spreader slide at a moderate speed toward the other end of the slide, keeping contact between the two slides at all times. Allow the slide to air dry before staining (Procedure 18-3).
Provides smooth movements and a thin film for viewing

7. Properly care for or dispose of equipment and supplies. Clean the work area. Wash your hands.

18

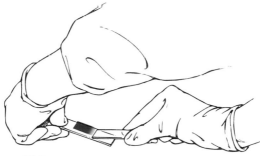

Figure 18-3. Hold spreader slide at a 30° angle and draw it back against the drop of blood.

Staining a Peripheral Blood Smear

Procedure Notes:

You Need to Know:

- An angle more or less than 30° provides an improper and possibly unreadable smear.
- Too much blood makes the smear invalid.
  (Note: See Procedure 18-2 for documentation guidelines and charting example.)

Before you begin to determine the types of WBCs on a slide, stain it this way.

Procedure 18-4

Staining a Peripheral Blood Smear

1. Assemble this equipment:
   - Staining rack
   - Wright stain
   - Buffer
   - Tweezers
   - Prepared slide

2. Follow these Standard Precautions.

3. Obtain a recently made and dried blood smear.
   Prevents specimen deterioration

4. Place the slide on a stain rack, blood side up.
   Provides stable surface for staining

5. Flood the slide with Wright stain. Allow the stain to remain on the slide for 3 to 5 minutes or for the time specified by the manufacturer.
   Fixes blood to slide and begins staining process

6. Using tweezers, tilt the slide so that the stain drains off. Apply buffer and then water in equal amounts. A green sheen will appear on the surface. Allow it to remain on

the slide for 5 minutes or the time specified by the manufacturer.

Provides buffers for Wright stain and enhances staining

7. Holding the slide with tweezers, gently rinse the slide
with water. Wipe off the back of the slide with gauze.
Stand the slide upright and allow it to dry before viewing (Procedure 18-4).

Rinses and removes excess stain for viewing under microscope

8. Properly care for or dispose of equipment and supplies.
Clean the work area. Wash your hands.

Procedure Notes:

You Need to Know:

• Some manufacturers provide a simple one-step method that consists of dipping the smear in a stain solution, then rinsing. Directions are provided by the manufacturer for this procedure and
vary with the specific test.

(Note: See Procedure 18-2 for documentation guidelines and
charting example.)

To determine the various types of WBCs in a smear, follow this procedure.

Procedure 18-5

Performing a WBC Differential

18

1. Assemble this equipment:
   • Stained peripheral blood smear
   • Microscope
   • Immersion oil
   • Paper
   • Recording tabulator

2. Follow these Standard Precautions.

3. Place the stained slide on the microscope. Focus on the feathered edge of the smear and scan to ensure an even distribution of cells and proper staining. Use the low-power objective.

4. Carefully turn nosepiece to high-power objective and bring into focus using the fine adjustment.
Allows visualization of slide

5. Place a drop of oil on the slide and rotate the oil immersion lens into place. Focus and begin to identify any leukocytes present.
Provides oil necessary for viewing

6. Record on a tally sheet or tabulator the types of WBCs found.
Ensures accuracy of percentages

7. Move the stage so that the next field is in view. Identify any WBCs in this field, and continue to the next field to identify all that are present until 100 WBCs have been counted.
Ensures that 100 cells have been counted

8. Calculate the number of each type of leukocyte as a percentage.
Provides proper percentage for comparison

9. Properly care for or dispose of equipment and supplies properly. Clean the work area. Wash your hands.

Procedure Notes:

18

You Need to Know:

- A WBC differential is performed by a trained laboratory technologist. Abnormal cells can appear in the peripheral blood; recognizing them is an important diagnostic procedure that requires specific training.
  (Note: See Procedure 18-1 for documentation guidelines and charting example.)

Does the physician suspect that your patient is anemic?

Procedure 18-6

Determining Hemoglobin Levels Using the Hemoglobinometer Method

1. Assemble this equipment:
   - Hemoglobinometer
   - Applicator sticks
   - Whole blood

2. Follow these Standard Precautions.

3. Obtain an EDTA (purple-topped tube) blood specimen from the patient, following the steps for capillary puncture described in Procedure 20-2.

4. Place a drop of well-mixed whole blood (obtained by venipuncture or skin puncture) on the glass chamber of hemoglobinometer. Place the coverslip over the chamber and slip the assembly into the holding clip.
   Prepares sample for hemoglobin determination

5. At one of the open edges, push the applicator stick into the chamber. Gently move the stick around until the specimen no longer appears cloudy.
   Lyses red cells; releases hemoglobin

6. Slide the chamber and clip assembly (clip) into the hemoglobinometer. If you are wearing a face shield, remove it now.
   Allows for color comparison reading

7. With your left hand, hold the meter and press the light button. View the field through the eyepiece. With your right hand, move the dial until both the right and left sides match each other in color intensity. Note the hemoglobin level indicated on the dial.
   Illuminates chamber to compare colors; matches fields to ensure accuracy of testing

18

Document on the Patient's Chart:

- Date and time
- Site of capillary puncture
- Type of test performed
- Performance of test
- Results of testing
- Action taken, if any
- Patient education and instructions
- Your signature

EXAMPLE

9/14/04	Pt. complained of having no energy.
9:45 AM	Periods have been heavy; pt. await-
	ing hysterectomy 10-1-04 for dys-
	functional bleeding. Cap puncture L
	ring finger. Hgb: 9.5. Dr. Royal noti-
	fied, ordered iron supplement.
	—C. Yamata, RMA

8. Clean the chamber and work area with 10% bleach solution. Dispose of equipment and supplies appropriately. Wash your hands.

18

Procedure Notes:

You Need to Know:

- Calibration chambers are included in the hemoglobinometer kit
  and are used to verify proper functioning of the meter. This procedure may vary according to the instrument used. Some manufacturers offer a digitally read hemoglobin device that is less subjective and is therefore considered more accurate and easier to use.

Does the physician suspect that a patient has anemia because of deficient RBCs? A microhematocrit is likely to be ordered.

Manual Microhematocrit Determination

1. Assemble this equipment:
   - Microcollection tubes
   - Sealing clay
   - Microhematocrit centrifuge
   - Microhematocrit reading device

2. Follow these Standard Precautions.

3. Draw blood into the capillary tube by one of two methods:

   a. Draw blood directly from a capillary puncture (Procedure 20-2) by touching the tip of the capillary tube to the blood at the puncture site and allowing it to fill ¾ of the tube or to the indicated mark.

   b. To take blood from a well-mixed anticoagulated (EDTA) tube or whole blood sample, touch the tip to the blood and allow it to fill ¾ of the tube.

4. Place your forefinger over the top of the tube, wipe excess blood off the sides, and push the bottom into the sealing clay. Draw a second specimen in the same manner.
   Anticoagulant prevents clotting; mixing well helps ensure accuracy.

5. Place the tubes opposite each other in the radial grooves of the microhematocrit centrifuge. Place the cover on top of the grooved area and tighten by turning the knob clockwise. Close the lid. Spin for 5 minutes, or as directed by the manufacturer.
   Balanced placement helps prevent damage to machine and ensures accuracy in testing.

6. Remove the tubes from the centrifuge and read the results from the reading device available (instructions are

18

Manual Microhematocrit Determination

Document on the Patient's Chart:

- Date and time
- Site of capillary puncture
- Type of test performed
- Performance of test
- Results of testing
- Action taken, if any
- Patient education and instructions
- Your signature

EXAMPLE

2/7/04	Capillary tube filled from skin punc-
1600	ture, left ring finger. Hct: 42%.
	Dr. Erickson notified.
	—Robin King, CMA

printed on the device). Results should be within 5% of each other. Take the average and report the result as a percentage. Some microhematocrit centrifuges have the scale printed within the machine at the radial grooves. *Identifies inappropriate results if they differ more than 5%*

7. Dispose of the microhematocrit tubes in a biohazard container. Properly care for or dispose of other equipment and supplies. Clean the work area. Wash your hands.

18

Procedure Notes:

You Need to Know:

- Some microhematocrit centrifuges have the scale printed within the machine at the radial grooves.

Need a nonspecific indicator of disease, such as inflammatory process? The physician may order a sed rate.

Procedure 18-8

Performing a Wintrobe ESR

1. Assemble this equipment:
   - Anticoagulation tube
   - Wintrobe tube
   - Transfer pipette
   - Timer

2. Follow these Standard Precautions.

3. Draw blood into an EDTA (purple-topped) anticoagulation tube.
   Prevents coagulation of specimen

4. Fill a graduated Wintrobe tube to the 0 mark with the well-mixed whole blood using the provided transfer pipette. Be sure to eliminate any trapped bubbles and fill exactly to the 0 line.
   Avoids altered test results

5. Place in a tube holder that allows the tube to remain straight up in a vertical position.

6. Wait exactly 1 hour; use a timer for accuracy. Keep the tube straight upright and undisturbed during the hour.
   Avoids altering results by tilting or disturbing tube

7. Record the level of the top of the red blood cells after 1 hour. Normal results for men are 0 to 10 mL/h; for women, 0 to 15 mL/h.

8. Properly care for or dispose of equipment and supplies. Clean the work area. Wash your hands.

Procedure Notes:

18

Document on the Patient's Chart:

- Date and time
- Site of venipuncture
- Performance of test
- Results of testing
- Action taken, if any
- Patient education and instructions
- Your signature

EXAMPLE

11/04/04	45-year-old woman presented with
1435	vague aches. Specimen drawn L an-
	tecubitus in purple-top tube per Dr.
	North's order. Wintrobe ESR test
	results 12 mL/h. Dr. North notified.
	—Sally Royal, CMA

You Need to Know:

- Never use a shorter time and multiply the reading; less time gives inaccurate results.

18 **This test aids in the evaluation of clotting disorders and determines the effectiveness of coagulation therapy.**

Procedure 18-9

Determining Bleeding Time

1. Assemble this equipment:
   - Blood pressure cuff
   - Autolet device

- Alcohol or antiseptic wipe
- Filter paper
- Butterfly bandage
- Stopwatch

2. Follow these Standard Precautions.

3. Position the patient so that the arm is extended in a manner that is both comfortable and stable.
   Helps ensure that patient does not move until procedure is complete

4. Have the patient turn the palm upward so that the inner aspect of the arm is exposed. Select a site several inches below the antecubital area. The area should be free of lesions and without visible veins. (The inner aspect provides a surface relatively free of hair.)

5. Apply the pressure cuff and set it at 40 mm Hg for the length of the test. Adjust it as needed throughout the test.
   Stabilizes the pressure to the arm

6. Twist the tear-away tab on the Autolet. Make an incision 1 mm in depth on the cleaned skin surface by placing the Autolet bleeding time device on the site and pressing the trigger button on the side. This releases the spring-loaded blade to make the incision. At the same time, start the stop watch.
   Disrupts surface capillaries but not underlying veins

7. At 30-second intervals, bring the filter paper near the edge of the wound to draw off some of the accumulating blood. Change the area of absorption on the filter paper each time. Avoid touching the wound with the filter paper.
   Provides area for observing the slowing of blood flow

8. The test is complete when the blood flow visibly stops. Stop the watch when no more blood is flowing; note the time. Remove pressure cuff.
   Indicates formation of platelet plug

18

Document on the Patient's Chart:

- Date and time
- Site of puncture
- Type of test performed
- Performance of test
- Results of test
- Action taken, if any
- Patient education and instructions
- Your signature

EXAMPLE

09/15/04	Skin puncture of L inner forearm,
1500	bleeding time test performed, re-
	sults 14 min. Dr. Lancaster notified.
	—Sam Goldstein, CMA

9. Apply a butterfly bandage across the wound to keep it sealed.
   Reduces scarring and protects wound

10. Properly care for or dispose of all equipment and supplies. Clean work area. Wash your hands.

Procedure Notes:

18

WARNING!

Be sure you are away from superficial veins. Puncturing superficial veins causes a prolonged bleeding time. If the patient is having clotting problems, excessive bleeding could occur.

You Need to Know:

- The filter paper should not touch the wound to avoid disruption of the platelet plug and an inaccurate measurement of bleeding time.

19

Microbiology

How do you keep a microscope in good working order?

Caring for a Microscope

1. Assemble this equipment:
   - Lens paper
   - Lens cleaner
   - Gauze
   - Mild soap solution
   - Microscope (Figure 19-1)

2. Follow these Standard Precautions.

3. Place a drop or two of lens cleaner on a piece of lens paper. Wipe each eyepiece thoroughly with the lens paper, then wipe each objective lens starting with the lowest power first and continuing to the highest power (usually an oil immersion lens). If at any time the lens paper appears to have dirt or oil on it, move to a clean section of the lens paper or use a new piece with cleaner to finish.

   Progresses from cleanest area (eyepieces) to least clean (oil immersion lens)

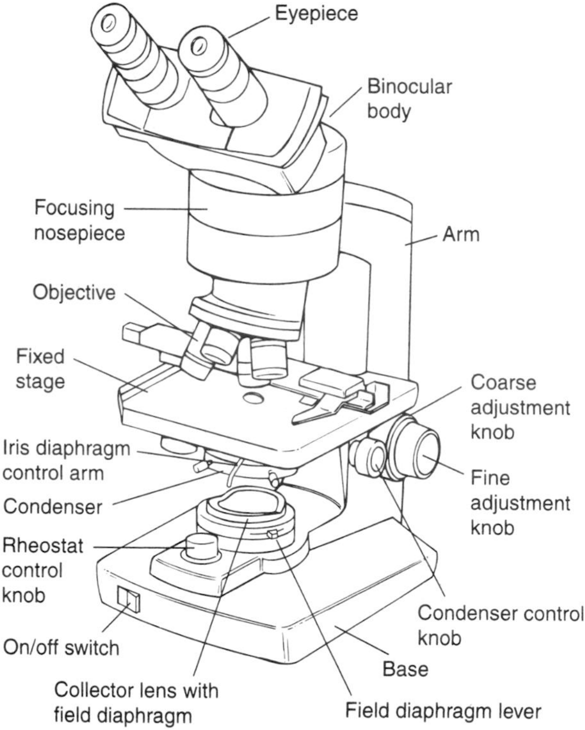

Figure 19-1. Standard light microscope.

4. Using a new piece of lens paper, wipe each eyepiece and objective so that no cleaner remains.
Prevents distortion caused by residue

5. Moisten gauze with mild soap and wipe down all nonocular areas (stage, base, adjustment knobs). Moisten another piece of gauze with water and rinse the washed areas.
Removes oil and dirt from mechanical and structural surfaces

6. Ensure that the light source is turned off. Rotate nosepiece so that the low-power objective is pointed down toward the stage. Cover the microscope if appropriate.
Protects mechanism and surfaces between uses

Procedure Notes:

- Read manufacturer's recommendations for proper care and cleaning of the microscope.
- To prevent scratches, never use tissue or gauze to clean ocular areas.
- To prevent the transfer of oils from your skin, do not touch ocular areas with your fingers.
- To change a light bulb, refer to the manufacturer's recommended procedures.
- Use two hands to carry the microscope, one to hold the base and the other to hold the arm.

How should a laboratory specimen be handled to ensure accurate test results?

Procedure 19-2

Preparing the Specimen for Transport

1. Assemble this equipment:
   - Appropriate laboratory requisition
   - Specimen container or mailing container
   - Specimen

2. Follow these Standard Precautions.

3. Complete the laboratory request form.
   Ensures that the test orders are correctly communicated

4. Check the expiration date and condition of the transport medium.
   Prevents use of out-of-date or compromised media

5. Peel the envelope away from the transport tube about ⅓ of the way and remove the tube.
   Provides for repackaging specimen

19

Preparing the Specimen for Transport

Document on the Patient's Chart:
- Date and time
- Site of collection
- Type of specimen
- Destination of specimen
- Your signature

EXAMPLE

7/13/04	Wound swab taken from left lower
1:00 PM	leg. Yellow-green drainage noted.
	Specimen was labeled and sent by
	courier to the laboratory.
	—Mark Thomas, RMA

6. Label the tube with the date, patient's name, source of the specimen, time of collection, and your initials.
Identifies specimen

7. Obtain the specimen as directed by the physician.
Ensures appropriate specimen for testing

8. Return the swab to the tube when appropriate and follow the manufacturer's recommendation for immersion into the medium. Package for transport as directed by the manufacturer.
Ensures proper growth or preservation conditions for specimen

9. Route the specimen.

19

Procedure Notes:

You Need to Know:
- Understand and follow the proper guidelines for collecting and handling specimens (Box 19-1).
- Be sure that any transport medium is free of contamination before using it. If the medium looks unusual in any way, do not use it.

BOX 19-1

Guidelines for Specimen Collection and Handling

- Follow Standard Precautions for specimen collection as outlined by the Centers for Disease Control and Prevention.
- Review the requirements for collecting and handling the specimen, including the equipment needed, the type of specimen to be collected (exudate, blood, mucus, and so on), the amount required for proper laboratory analysis, and the procedure to be followed for handling and storage.
- Assemble the equipment and supplies. Use only the appropriate specimen container for the sample to be submitted as specified by the medical office or laboratory.
- Ensure that the specimen container is sterile to prevent contamination of the specimen by organisms not present at the collection site.
- Examine each container before use to make sure that it is not damaged, the medium is intact and moist, and it is well within the expiration date.
- Label each tube or specimen container with the patient's name and/or identification number, the date, the name or initials of the person collecting the specimen, the source or site of the specimen, and any other information required by the laboratory. Use an indelible pen or permanent marker. Make sure you print legibly, document accurately, and include all pertinent information.

19

- Be aware that some transport medium requires special storage, such as refrigeration.
- Follow quality control (QC) measures, such as these:
  —Dating medium when it is received
  —Rotating stock with oldest in front
  —Recording lot numbers and expiration dates on a QC log in the laboratory

Preparing a Dry Smear

Instruct the Patient Regarding:

- Test name (e.g., blood cell count, occult blood)
- Specimen type required (e.g., blood, urine, stool)
- Reason for test
- Directions for proper collection, handling, and storage if specimen is to be collected at home

Do you need to prepare a slide for identification of pathogenic bacteria?

Procedure 19-3

Preparing a Dry Smear

1. Assemble this equipment:
   - Specimen
   - Slide forceps
   - Sterile swab or inoculating loop
   - Bunsen burner
   - Slide
   - Pencil or diamond-tipped pen

2. Follow these Standard Precautions.

3. Label the slide with the patient's name, date, and specimen source on the frosted edge. Use pencil or diamond-tipped pen.
   Provides proper identification

19

4. Hold the edges of the slide between the thumb and index finger. Starting at the right side of the slide and using a rolling motion of the swab or a sweeping motion of the inoculating loop, gently and evenly spread the material from the specimen over the slide (Figure 19-2). The material should thinly fill the center of the slide within ½ inch of each end.
   Avoids obscuring slide with too much material

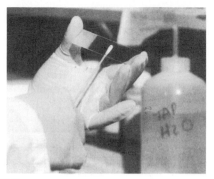

Figure 19-2. Spread the material from the specimen over the slide.

5. Dispose of the contaminated swab or inoculating loop in a biohazard container. If you are not using a disposable loop, sterilize it as follows:

    a. Hold the loop in the colorless part of the flame of the Bunsen burner for 10 seconds.

    b. Raise the loop slowly (to avoid splattering the bacteria) to the blue part of the flame until the loop and its connecting wire glow red.

    c. If reusing the loop, cool the loop so the heat does not kill the bacteria that must be allowed to grow. Do not wave the loop in the air because doing so may expose it to contamination. Do not stab the medium with a hot loop to cool. This creates an aerosol.
    Prevents exposure to biohazardous material, preserves integrity of specimen

6. Allow the smear to air dry in a flat position for at least ½ hour. Note: Some specimens require a fixative spray (e.g., Pap smears).
Keeps cells from becoming distorted

7. Hold the dried smear slide with the slide forceps. Pass the slide quickly through the flame of a Bunsen burner three or four times. The slide has been fixed properly when the back of the slide feels uncomfortably warm to the back of the hand. It should not feel hot.
Fixes specimen to slide

19

Preparing a Dry Smear

Document on the Patient's Chart:
- Date and time
- Site of collection
- Type of specimen
- Results of testing, if applicable
- Action taken, if any
- Patient education and instructions
- Your signature

EXAMPLE

8/12/04	Specimen taken from nasal cavity
8:30 AM	and prepared as a dry smear.
	Gram-positive cocci in clusters.
	Dr. York read the slide.
	—T. Diaz, CMA

8. Examine the smear under the microscope or stain it according to office policy. In most instances, the physician examines the slide for identification.

9. Dispose of equipment and supplies in appropriate containers. Clean the work area. Wash your hands.
Prevents the spread of microorganisms

Procedure Notes:

19

You Need to Know:
- Do not rub material vigorously over the slide; this may destroy fragile organisms.
- Do not wave the slide in the air; this could cause contamination.
- Do not apply heat until the specimen has been allowed to dry.
- Spray fixatives immediately and from a distance of 4 to 6 inches to protect the cells from contaminants or to keep them from becoming dislodged.

Instruct the Patient Regarding:

- Proper collection of male urethral smear:
  - —In the restroom, expose the penis and allow a small portion of discharge to touch the slide
  - —Do not wash the end of the penis before collecting the specimen; doing so washes away organisms that may be present
  - —Bring the slide to the laboratory
- Caution the patient to wash his hands well and practice proper personal hygiene

Note: Medical assistants should wear PPE to receive and handle the slide.

After preparing the dry slide, how should you stain it to identify the microorganism?

Procedure 19-4

Gram Staining a Smear Slide

1. Assemble this equipment:
   - Crystal violet stain
   - Gram iodine solution
   - Alcohol-acetone solution
   - Counterstain (e.g., safranin)
   - Specimen on a glass slide labeled using a diamond-tipped pen
   - Bunsen burner
   - Slide forceps
   - Staining rack
   - Wash bottle with distilled water
   - Absorbent (bibulous) paper pad
   - Immersion oil
   - Microscope
   - Stopwatch or timer

2. Follow these Standard Precautions.

3. Make sure that the specimen is heat-fixed to the labeled side and that the slide is at room temperature before beginning (see Procedure 19-3: Preparing a Dry Smear).

19

4. Place the slide on the staining rack with the smear side upward.
Ensures collection of dye as it runs off slide for disposal

5. Flood the smear with crystal violet stain. Time immersion with the stopwatch or timer for 30 or 60 seconds.
Stains bacteria purple

6. Hold the slide with slide forceps.

   a. Tilt the slide to a 45° angle to drain the excess dye.

   b. Rinse the slide with distilled water from the wash bottle for about 5 seconds, and drain off the excess water.
   Stops the coloring process

7. Replace the slide on the slide rack. Flood the slide with Gram iodine solution, and time the process for 30 or 60 seconds.
Acts as a mordant and fixes, or binds, crystal violet stain

8. Using the forceps, tilt the slide at a 45° angle to drain the iodine solution. With the slide tilted, rinse the slide with distilled water from the wash bottle for about 5 seconds. Slowly and gently wash with the alcohol-acetone solution until no more purple stain runs off (5 to 10 seconds).
Removes crystal violet stain from the Gram-negative bacteria; Gram-positive bacteria retain purple dye

9. Immediately rinse the slide with distilled water for 5 seconds, and return the slide to the rack.
Stops decolorizing process

10. Flood with the safranin or a suitable counterstain. Time process for 30 or 60 seconds.
Stains Gram-negative bacteria pink or red with counterstain

11. Drain the excess counterstain from the slide by tilting it at a 45° angle.

    a. Rinse the slide with the distilled water for 5 seconds to remove the counterstain.
    Prevents obscuring slide and aids identification

    b. Gently blot the smear dry using absorbent bibulous paper. Take care not to disturb the smeared specimen. Wipe the back of the slide clear of any solution.

19

12. Inspect slide, using oil immersion objective lens for greater magnification. The physician interprets the slide. Figure 19-3 shows various morphologies of bacteria.

13. Properly care for or dispose of equipment and supplies. Clean the work area. Wash your hands.
    Prevents spread of microorganisms

Procedure Notes:

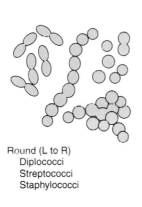

Round (L to R)
  Diplococci
  Streptococci
  Staphylococci

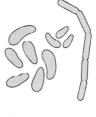

Rod-shaped
  Bacilli
  or
  Coccobacilli

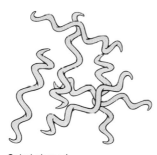

Spiral-shaped
  Spirochetes

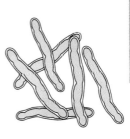

Curved rods
  Spirilla
  Vibrios

Figure 19-3. Morphology of bacteria.

> **WARNING!**
> · Be consistent with the times. If you use 30 seconds, use it throughout the procedure.
> · If the decolorizing process is carried on too long or too vigorously, dye may leach out of the Gram-positive bacteria and lead to incorrect test results.

You Need to Know:

- Results may be misinterpreted if the reagents are defective or near expiration, or if the timing factors in the staining process are not as directed.
- The bacteria may be overstained or may have color leached from the cells if care is not taken to observe the time limits.
- The results are not accurate if the specimen is not heated properly (causing the bacteria to die) or is not incubated long enough, or if the general technique is not performed correctly.
- Prepared smears of known Gram-positive and Gram-negative organisms are processed with the patient's specimen for quality control.
- Labeling the slide with a diamond-tipped pen ensures that the identification does not wash off during the repeated staining and washing steps of the procedure.
  (Note: See Procedure 19-2 for documentation guidelines and charting example.)

How should you prepare a culture medium to promote the growth of pathogens and to identify microorganisms?

Procedure 19-5

19

Inoculating a Culture

1. Assemble this equipment:
   - Specimen on a swab or in proper container
   - China marker or permanent laboratory markers
   - Inoculating loop
   - Bunsen burner
   - Labeled Petri dish

2. Follow these Standard Precautions.

3. Label the plate, on the bottom of the medium side, with the patient's name, identification number, source of specimen, time collected, time inoculated, your initials, and date.
Ensures that plate is read at proper time

4. Remove the cover from the Petri plate and place it with the opening upward on the work surface. Do not open the cover unnecessarily.
Reduces possibility of contamination

5. Using a rolling and sliding motion, streak the specimen swab completely across half of the plate starting from the top and working to a midpoint or at the diameter of the plate. Dispose of the swab in a biohazard container.
Spreads specimen in gradually thinning colonies

6. If your office does not use disposable inoculating loops, sterilize the loop as described in step 5 of Procedure 19-3: Preparing a Dry Smear.

7. Turn the plate ¼ turn from its previous position. Pass the loop a few times in the original inoculum and then into half of the remaining uninoculated medium, streaking approximately ¼ of the surface of the plate (Figure 19-4). Do not enter the originally streaked area after the first few sweeps.
Draws bits of specimen into clean surface

8. Turn the plate another ¼ turn. Working in the previous manner, draw the loop through the most recently streaked area once or twice. Do not enter the originally streaked area. Replace cover.
Pulls out gradually thinning bits of specimen to isolate colonies; provides for easier identification

9. Properly care for or dispose of equipment and supplies. Clean work area. Wash your hands.
Prevents spread of microorganisms

19

Inoculating a Culture

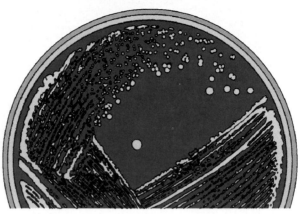

Figure 19-4. A properly prepared culture plate after incubation.

10. Incubate for the specified period of time. Read the results and record as directed by office policy. (Never use a shorter time and multiply the reading; less time gives inaccurate results.)

Procedure Notes:

You Need to Know:

- For sensitivity and quantity identification, use the same procedure and supplies. The method of distribution differs by streaking the inoculate (specimen) down the center of the plate and spreading it across the entire surface of the medium using a sterile loop.
- Using sterile forceps or an automatic dispenser, place the specified medication disks on areas of the plate equidistant from each other. Press them gently with the sterilized loop or forceps until good contact is made with the surface of the medium.

Document on the Patient's Chart:

* Date and time
* Site of specimen
* Performance of test
* Results of test at appropriate time
* Action taken, if any
* Patient education and instructions
* Your signature

EXAMPLE

7/14/04	Swab specimen taken of (L) heel
0915	wound, transferred to culture
	medium for incubation. To be read
	07/16/04. Pt. instructed on wound
	care and infection control; verbal-
	ized understanding of instructions.
	—Karen Glass, CMA
7/16/04	Specimen checked by Dr. Persons.
0830	Pt. instructed to RTC today for
	wound débridement and further
	treatment.
	—Karen Glass, CMA

19

20

Phlebotomy

Do you need to draw blood from a patient for testing?

Procedure 20-1

Obtaining a Blood Specimen by Venipuncture

1. Assemble this equipment:
   - Needle, syringe, and tube(s) or evacuated tubes
   - Tourniquet
   - Sterile gauze pads
   - Bandages
   - Needle and adapter
   - Sharps container
   - 70% alcohol pad or alternate antiseptic
   - Permanent marker or pen

2. Follow these Standard Precautions.

3. Check the requisition slip to determine the tests ordered and specimen requirements.
   Ensures proper specimen collection

4. Check the expiration date on the tubes. Be aware that certain tube colors have specific uses (Table 20-1).

5. Greet and identify the patient. Explain the procedure. Ask for and answer any questions.

Table 20-1

Evacuated Tube System: Color Coding

Tube Color	Additive	Laboratory Use
Purple	Ethylenediaminete-traacetic acid (EDTA)	Hematology testing
Blue	Sodium citrate	Coagulation studies (fill to proper level)
Green	Lithium heparin or sodium heparin	Blood gases and pH; cytogenetics
Gray	Potassium oxalate or sodium fluoride	Glucose testing
Red	None	Serum testing
Red/yellow	Glass particles	Chemistry
Red/gray	Thixotropic gel	Chemistry

6. If a fasting specimen is required, ask the patient when she last had anything to eat or drink.
   Ensures accuracy of results

7. Put on gloves.
   Protects against exposure to biohazardous material

8. Break the seal of the needle cover and thread the sleeved needle into the adapter, using the needle cover as a wrench. Tap the tubes that contain additives to ensure that the additive is dislodged from the stopper and wall of the tube. Insert the tube into the adapter until the needle slightly enters the stopper. Do not push the top of the tube stopper beyond the indentation mark. If the tube retracts slightly, leave it in the retracted position. If using a syringe, tighten the needle on the hub and "breathe" the syringe.
   Ensures proper needle placement and tube positioning, and prevents loss of vacuum or sticking of plunger in syringe barrel

9. Have the patient sit in a position that ensures a well-supported arm, with the arm in a downward extended, slightly flexed position if possible.

20

10. Apply the tourniquet around the patient's arm 3 to 4 inches above the elbow.
Causes distal vasodilation for proper site identification and easier venous access

11. Apply the tourniquet snugly, but not too tightly.
Promotes patient comfort

12. Secure the tourniquet by using the half-bow.
Allows for easy removal

13. Make sure the tails of the tourniquet extend upward to avoid contaminating the venipuncture site.

14. Ask the patient to close her hand into a fist, but ask her not to pump her fist.
Raises the vessels out of underlying tissues and muscles

15. Select a vein (see Figure 9-4) by palpating. Use your gloved index finger to trace the path of the vein and judge its depth.
Provides most sensitive area for palpation

16. Release the tourniquet after palpating the vein if it has been left on for more than 1 minute.

17. Cleanse the venipuncture site with an alcohol pad starting in the center of puncture site and working outward in a circular motion.
Avoids recontamination of area

18. Reapply the tourniquet if it was removed after palpation.
Prevents altered test results

19. Remove the needle cover. Hold the syringe or evacuated assembly in your dominant hand. Your thumb should be on top of the adapter and your fingers underneath. Grasp the patient's arm with the nondominant hand while using your thumb to draw the skin taut over the site and anchor the vein about 1 to 2 inches below the puncture site.
Anchoring allows for easier needle penetration and less pain

20. With the bevel up, line up the needle with the vein approximately $\frac{1}{4}$ to $\frac{1}{2}$ inch below the site where the vein is to be entered. At a 15° to 30° angle, rapidly and smoothly insert the needle through the skin (Figure 20-1).

20

21. Remove your nondominant hand and slowly pull back the plunger of the syringe, or place two fingers on the flanges of the adapter, and with the thumb push the tube onto the needle inside the adapter. When blood begins to flow into the tube or syringe, release the tourniquet and allow the patient to release the fist. Allow the syringe or tube(s) to fill to capacity. When blood flow ceases, remove the tube from the adapter by gripping the tube with your nondominant hand, and place your thumb against the flange during removal.

22. Gently pull out the tube. If the tube contains an additive, immediately invert it 5 to 10 times.
    Allows for mixing additives and blood

23. Steady the needle in the vein. To prevent discomfort, try not to pull up or press down on the needle while it is in the vein. Insert any other necessary tubes into the adapter and allow it to fill to capacity.

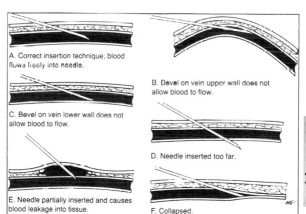

A. Correct insertion technique; blood flows freely into needle.

B. Bevel on vein upper wall does not allow blood to flow.

C. Bevel on vein lower wall does not allow blood to flow.

D. Needle inserted too far.

E. Needle partially inserted and causes blood leakage into tissue.

F. Collapsed.

Figure 20-1. Proper and improper needle positioning. **(A)** Proper needle position. **(B)** Needle bevel against the upper wall of a vein. **(C)** Needle bevel against or embedded in opposite wall of vein. **(D)** Needle inserted all the way through a vein. **(E)** Needle partially inserted into a vein. **(F)** Needle in collapsed vein.

20

24. Remove the tube from the adapter before removing the needle from the arm. If the tourniquet has not been previously released, do so now.
Prevents blood from dripping on patient or assistant

25. Place a sterile gauze pad over the puncture site at the time of needle withdrawal. Do not apply any pressure to the site until the needle is completely removed.
Prevents patient discomfort; protects wound

26. After the needle is removed, apply pressure or have the patient apply direct pressure for 3 to 5 minutes.
Assists with coagulation at site

27. Transfer the blood from the syringe into the proper tube by inserting the needle through the stopper and allowing the vacuum to pull blood into the tubes. Use proper "order of draw" (Table 20-2).
Prevents clotting of blood

28. Label the tubes with the proper information.
Provides proper identification

29. Check the puncture site for bleeding. Apply a bandage.
Protects wound site

30. Properly care for or dispose of all equipment and supplies. Clean the work area. Wash your hands.
Ensures that equipment and supplies are available for next use; prevents spread of microorganisms

31. Test, transfer, or store the blood specimen according to medical office policy.

Procedure Notes:

20

WARNING!

· *In the event that you accidentally enter an artery, keep pressure on the site for a minimum of 5 minutes. Note it on the patient's chart.*
· *Never release a patient until bleeding has stopped.*
· *When transferring blood from a syringe to a tube, do not hold the tube when puncturing the stopper and filling the tube; place it in a tube rack and carefully insert the needle through the stopper.*

Table 20-2

Order of Draw

Evacuated Tube System

- Blood culture tubes (and other tests requiring sterile specimens)
- Red stopper or red/gray stopper (nonadditive and gel separator)
- Light blue stopper (if light blue stoppered tube is the first and only tube to be drawn, draw a 5-mL, red-stopper tube first and discard it to eliminate contamination from tissue thromboplastin picked up during needle penetration)
- Green stopper
- Purple stopper
- Gray stopper

Syringe System

- Blood culture
- Light blue stopper
- Purple stopper
- Green stopper
- Gray stopper
- Red stopper

You Need to Know:

- Puncturing a wet area stings, causes hemolysis of the sample, and may interfere with some test results. Allow the site to dry or dry the site with sterile gauze. Do not touch the area after cleansing.
- If the blood is being used for diagnosing septic conditions, make sure the specimen is sterile. To do this, apply alcohol to the area for 2 full minutes. Then apply a 2% iodine solution in ever-widening circles. Never move the wipes back over areas that have been cleaned; use a new wipe for each sweep across the area.
- Tourniquets should not be left on for more than 1 minute at a time during this procedure.
- Removing the tourniquet during the draw releases pressure on the vein and helps prevent blood from seeping into adjacent tissues and causing a hematoma.

20

Document on the Patient's Chart:

- Date and time
- Site of venipuncture
- Performance of procedure
- Patient observations
- Routing of specimen or on-site testing results
- Patient education and instructions
- Your signature

EXAMPLE

4/5/04	Venipuncture to left forearm. Three
1330	collection tubes filled. Tubes la-
	beled and sent to Met-path labs.
	Pt. tolerated procedure well.
	—William Gray, CMA

- When the procedure is complete, do not have the patient bend the arm at the elbow. Bending the arm increases the chance of blood seeping into the subcutaneous tissues.
- If the vacuum tubes contain an anticoagulant, they must be mixed immediately by gently inverting the tube 8 to 10 times. Do not shake the tube.

Instruct the Patient to:

- Apply pressure to the site to decrease the amount of blood escaping into the tissues

20

Do you need a small amount of your patient's blood for testing?

Procedure 20-2

Obtaining a Blood Specimen by Skin Puncture

1. Assemble this equipment:
   - Sterile disposable lancet or automated skin puncture device
   - 70% alcohol or alternate antiseptic
   - Sterile gauze pads
   - Collection containers (Unopette, capillary tubes)
   - Heel-warming device, if needed

2. Follow these Standard Precautions.

3. Check the requisition slip to determine the tests ordered and specimen requirements.
   Ensures proper specimen collection

4. Greet and identify the patient. Explain the procedure. Ask for and answer any questions.

5. Put on gloves.

6. Select the puncture site (the lateral portion of the tip of the middle or ring finger of the nondominant hand, lateral curved surface of the heel, or great toe of an infant). Make the puncture in the fleshy, central portion of the second or third finger, slightly to the side of center and perpendicular to the grooves of the fingerprint (Figure 20-2). Perform heel puncture only on the plantar surface of the heel, medial to an imaginary line extending from the middle of the great toe to the heel, or lateral to an imaginary line drawn from between the fourth and fifth toes to the heel (Figure 20-3). Puncture should not exceed 2.4 mm in depth.

7. Gently massage the finger from the base to the tip, or warm the site for 3 minutes with a warm washcloth or commercial heel warmer.
   Increases local vasodilation

20

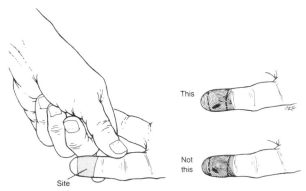

This

Not this

Site

Figure 20-2. Recommended site and direction of finger puncture.

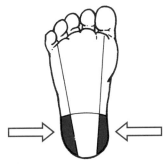

Figure 20-3. Acceptable areas for heel-skin punctures on newborn infants.

20

8. Grasp the finger firmly between your nondominant index finger and the thumb, or grasp the infant's heel firmly with the index finger wrapped around the foot and the thumb wrapped around the ankle. Cleanse the ball of the selected finger or heel with 70% isopropyl alcohol, and wipe dry with a sterile gauze pad or allow to air dry.

Prevents contaminating cleansed puncture area; allows control of puncture site

9. Hold the patient's finger or heel firmly and make a swift, deep puncture. Perform the puncture perpendicular to the whorls of the fingerprint or footprint.
Allows blood to form rounded drop for easier collection

   a. Always wipe away the first drop of blood with a sterile dry gauze.
   Prevents contamination of specimen

   b. Apply pressure toward the site but do not "milk" the site.
   Prevents dilution of specimen by tissue fluid

10. Collect the required specimen in the chosen containers or slides. Do not touch the collection device to the puncture site to avoid contaminating the wound. Touch only the tip of the device to the drop of blood to prevent contaminating inappropriate parts of the device.

11. When collection is complete, apply pressure to the site with clean gauze until bleeding stops.

12. Label the containers with the proper information.
Identifies specimen

13. Properly care for or dispose of equipment and supplies. Clean the work area. Wash your hands.

14. Test, transfer, or store the blood specimen according to the medical office policy.

Procedure Notes:

WARNING!

20

· Do not apply bandages to skin punctures of infants under 2 years of age. Younger children may develop a skin irritation from the adhesive bandage. Also, a young child might aspirate the bandage and choke.
· Never release a patient until bleeding has stopped.

Obtaining a Blood Specimen by Skin Puncture

Document on the Patient's Chart:

- Date and time
- Site of puncture
- Performance of testing
- Action taken, if any
- Routing of specimen, if appropriate
- Patient education and instructions
- Your signature

EXAMPLE

2/7/04	Capillary puncture to right ring fin-
3:00 PM	ger. Blood collected in microcollec-
	tion tube.
	—R. Jones, RMA

You Need to Know:

- The ring and middle fingers are less calloused and the lateral part of the tip is the least sensitive part of the finger.
- A puncture made across the contours of the fingerprint produces a large, round drop of blood.
- In an infant skin puncture, the area and the depth designated reduce the risk of puncturing the bone.
- Make sure the site chosen is warm and not cyanotic or edematous. Blood flow is encouraged if the puncture site is held in a downward, or dependent, angle and gentle pressure is applied to the site.
- Scraping the collection device on the skin activates platelets and may cause hemolysis.
- Mixing the specimens prevents clotting.
- Cap microcollection tubes with the caps provided, and mix the additives by gently tilting or inverting the tubes 8 to 10 times.

20

Urinalysis

**Is a patient complaining of urinary symptoms?
Use this method to obtain a specimen.**

Procedure 21-1

**Obtaining a Clean Catch Midstream (CCMS) Urine
Specimen**

1. Assemble this equipment:
   - Sterile cotton balls or appropriate antiseptic wipes
   - Antiseptic (if using cotton balls)
   - Sterile water
   - Sterile urine container labeled with patient's name
   - Bedpan or urinal (if necessary)

2. Follow these Standard Precautions.

3. Identify the patient and explain the procedure. Ask for
   and answer any questions.

4. If the patient is to perform the procedure, provide the
   necessary supplies.

5. Have the patient perform the procedure.

   a. Instruct the male patient to do the following:

      (1) Expose the glans penis by retracting the fore-
          skin, then clean the meatus with an antiseptic
          wipe or a cotton ball soaked in a mild antiseptic.

Clean the glans in a circular motion away from the meatus. Use a new wipe for each cleaning sweep.

Removes microorganisms from the urinary meatus and surrounding skin

(2) Keeping the foreskin retracted, void the first portion, about 30 mL, into the toilet or urinal.

Washes away organisms in the lower urethra and at the meatus

(3) Bring the sterile container into the urine stream and collect a sufficient amount (about 30 to 100 mL). Avoid touching the inside of the container with the penis.

Prevents specimen contamination

(4) Finish voiding into the toilet or urinal.

Avoids contamination of specimen by prostatic fluid

b. Instruct the female patient to do the following:

(1) Kneel or squat over a bedpan or toilet bowl. Spread the labia minora widely to expose the meatus. Using an antiseptic wipe or cotton balls soaked in a mild antiseptic, cleanse on either side of the meatus, then the meatus itself. Use a wipe or cotton ball only once in a sweep from the anterior to the posterior surfaces, then discard it. Rinse with cotton balls soaked in sterile water in the same manner.

Removes microorganisms from the urinary meatus

(2) Keeping the labia separated, void the first portion, about 30 mL, into the toilet.

Washes away organisms remaining in the meatus

(3) Bring the sterile container into the urine stream and collect a sufficient amount (about 30 to 100 mL).

(4) Finish voiding into the toilet or bedpan. Do not touch the inside of the container.

Touching the inside of the container may cause contamination

21

Document on the Patient's Chart:

- Date and time
- Performance of procedure
- Physical observations
- Chemical testing results
- Action taken (if any)
- Patient education and instructions
- Your signature

EXAMPLE

11/09/04	Pt. instructed in cleansing proce-
1630	dure and midstream collection of
	urine. Urine specimen collected and
	labeled. Color: straw; clarity: clear;
	specific gravity, tested with uri-
	nometer: 1.020; dipstick was nega-
	tive; pH: 7.0.
	—Gene Daggle, RMA

6. Cap the filled container, and drop it into the outer carrying container or place it in a designated area.
Prevents exposure to biohazardous material

7. Properly care for or dispose of equipment and supplies. Clean the work area. Wash your hands.
Ensures a clean work environment; prevents spread of microorganisms

Procedure Notes:

21

WARNING!

Some antiseptic wipes may interfere with protein testing. Note the type of antiseptic used on the patient's chart.

Obtaining a 24-Hour Urine Specimen

You Need to Know:

- Patients who are physically limited may need assistance in collecting the specimen.

Instruct the Patient Regarding:

- Collecting a sample from the middle of the urine stream ensures the least contamination with skin bacteria.

When a quantitative urinalysis is needed, the specimen is collected over a 24-hour period.

Procedure 21-2

Obtaining a 24-Hour Urine Specimen

1. Assemble this equipment:
   - Patient's labeled 24-hour urine container (some patients may require more than one container)
   - Preservatives required for the specific test
   - Hazard labels
   - Volumetric cylinder (holds at least 1 liter)
   - Serologic or volumetric pipettes
   - Clean urine container
   - Fresh 10% bleach solution
   - Patient log form

2. Follow these Standard Precautions.

3. Identify the type of 24-hour urine collection requested and check for any special requirements, such as any acid or preservative that should be added. Label the container appropriately.
   Additives protect the integrity of the specimen.

4. Put on gloves and PPE gown.

5. Add to the 24-hour urine container the correct amount of acid or preservative, if needed, using a serologic or volumetric pipette.
   Prevents altered testing results caused by incorrect preparation

21

6. Use a label provided or write on the 24-hour urine container "Beginning Time _____ and Date _____" and "Ending Time _____ and Date _____" so that the patient can fill in the appropriate information.
Documents testing times

7. Instruct the patient to collect a 24-hour urine sample as follows:

   a. Void into the toilet and note this time and date as the beginning.

   b. After the first voiding, collect each voiding and add it to the urine container for the next 24 hours.

   c. Precisely 24 hours after beginning collection, empty the bladder even if there is no urge to void and add this to the container.

   d. Note on the label the ending time and date.

8. Explain to the patient that, depending on the test requested, the 24-hour urine sample may need to be refrigerated the entire time. Instruct the patient to return the specimen to you as soon as possible after collection is complete.
Prevents degradation of urine components, which can alter results

9. Record in the patient's chart that supplies and instructions were given to collect a 24-hour urine specimen and the test that was requested.
Documents patient education and instructions

10. After receiving the 24-hour urine specimen from the patient, verify beginning and ending times and dates before the patient leaves. Check for required acids or preservatives that need to be added before routing the specimen to the laboratory, if applicable.
Protects integrity of specimen

11. Pour the urine into a cylinder to record the total volume collected during the 24-hour period. Pour a small representative sample (aliquot) of the urine into a clean container to be sent to the laboratory. Record the volume of the urine collection and the amount of acid or preservative added (if needed) on the sample container

21

and on the laboratory requisition. If permissible, you may dispose of the remainder of the urine.
Adheres to testing protocol

12. Record the volume on the patient log form.

13. Clean the cylinder with fresh 10% bleach solution, then rinse with water. Let it air dry.

14. Clean the work area and dispose of waste properly. Remove PPE gown and wash your hands.
Ensures a clean work environment; prevents spread of microorganisms

Procedure Notes:

WARNING!

Use caution when handling acids or other types of hazardous materials. Be familiar with the Material Safety Data Sheets (MSDSs) for each chemical at your site.

You Need to Know:

- Depending on the type of office and laboratory in which you work, you may not need to remove an aliquot of the 24-hour urine specimen.
- Label the specimen with a biohazard label if this is not prominently displayed on the container.

Instruct the Patient or Caregiver Regarding:

- Proper collection procedure
- Importance of collecting all voided urine during the collection period

21

Document on the Patient's Chart:

- Date and time
- Performance of procedure
- Testing results
- Action taken
- Patient education and instructions
- Your signature

EXAMPLE

3/8/04	Pt. instructed to collect urine for
0930	24 hours. Pt. was given container
	and written instructions. Pt. to
	begin collecting at 8:00 AM on 3/9
	and to end at 8:00 AM on 3/10.
	Will bring specimen in on 3/10.
3/10/04	Pt. returned with completed 24-
1010	hour specimen collection. Total
	volume = 1,850 mL. Labeled
	50-mL aliquot sent to Control
	Path Lab.
	—Tom Killet, CMA

21

Determining Color and Clarity of Urine

The color and clarity of urine are important indicators of health.

Procedure 21-3

Determining Color and Clarity of Urine

1. Assemble this equipment:
   - Patient's labeled urine specimen
   - Clear glass tube, usually a centrifuge tube
   - White paper scored with black lines

2. Follow these Standard Precautions.

3. Wash your hands and put on gloves, PPE gown, and face shield.

4. Verify that the names on the specimen container and the laboratory form are the same.
   Avoids errors in identification

5. Pour 10 to 15 mL of urine into the tube.
   Provides an adequate quantity for testing

6. In bright light, examine the urine for color. Record color on laboratory form.
   Provides illumination for testing; complies with documentation guidelines

7. Hold the urine tube in front of the white paper scored with black lines to determine clarity (Figure 21-1).
   Provides standard for clarity comparison

8. If the lines are seen clearly (not obscured), record as clear. If the lines are seen but are not well delineated, record as hazy. If the lines cannot be seen at all, record as cloudy.
   Provides consistency in reporting

9. Properly care for or dispose of equipment and supplies. If further urine testing is required, cover or cap tube.
   Protects integrity of specimen

21

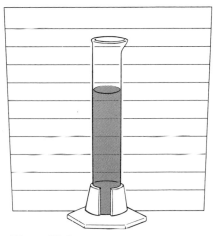

Figure 21-1. Observe the urine for clarity.

10. Clean the work area. Remove gloves, gown, and shield. Wash your hands.

Ensures a clean work environment; prevents the spread of pathogens

Procedure Notes:

You Need to Know:

- The most common colors are straw (very pale yellow), yellow, dark yellow, and amber. See Table 21-1 for an explanation of urine colors and possible causes.
- Rapid determination of color and clarity are necessary because some urine turns cloudy if left standing.
- Bilirubin, which may be found in urine in certain conditions, breaks down when exposed to light. Protect the specimen from light if urinalysis is ordered but testing is delayed.
- If further testing is to be done but is delayed, refrigerate the specimen to avoid alteration of urine chemistry levels.

21

Determining Color and Clarity of Urine

Table 21-1

Common Causes for Variations in the Color and Clarity of Urine

Color or Clarity	Possible Causes
Yellow-brown or green-brown	Bile in urine (as in jaundice), phenol poisoning (also known as carbolic acid, used as an antimicrobial agent)
Dark yellow or orange	Concentrated urine, low fluid intake, dehydration, inability of kidney to dilute urine, fluorescein (an intravenous dye), excessive carotene (carotenemia)
Bright orange-red	Pyridium (a urinary tract analgesic)
Red or reddish-brown	Fresh blood (indicating bleeding in the lower urinary tract), porphyrin menstrual contamination (porphyrin binds with iron to form heme), pyrvinium pamoate for intestinal worms, sulfonamides (sulfa-based antibiotics)
Brownish-black	Methylene blue medication (commonly used as an antiseptic or in the treatment of a form of anemia)
Black	Melanin (cell pigment)
Grayish or smoky	Hemoglobin or remnants of old RBC (indicating bleeding in the upper urinary tract), chyle, prostatic fluid, yeasts
Cloudy	Phosphate precipitation (normal after sitting for a prolonged time), urate (a compound of uric acid), leukocytes, pus, blood, epithelial cells, fat droplets, strict vegetarian diet

Note: In addition to the causes noted above, foods such as blackberries, rhubarb, beets, and those with red dye are common causes of dark or reddish urine that might resemble hematuria.

21

Document on the Patient's Chart:

- Date and time
- Performance of procedure
- Testing results
- Action taken (if any)
- Your signature

EXAMPLE

3/8/04	Random urine collected. Yellow,
1105	clear. Urine dip negative for glucose
	and protein.
	—Sam Pell, RMA

The specific gravity of urine can be determined by refractometer testing.

Procedure 21-4

Determining Specific Gravity (SG) of Urine Using a Refractometer

1. Assemble this equipment:
   - Patient's labeled urine specimen
   - Transfer pipettes
   - Refractometer
   - Wipe or clean gauze
   - Light source

2. Follow these Standard Precautions.

21

3. Verify that the names on the specimen container and the laboratory form are the same.

4. Wash your hands and put on PPE gown, gloves, and face shield.

5. Make sure the refractometer is clean before beginning. Use distilled water and a wipe or gauze to wipe the cover and the prism so they are clean and free of moisture.

6. Using a clean pipette, place a drop of the patient's well-mixed, room-temperature urine onto the notch of the cover. The urine should flow over the prism.
Delivers the specimen for reading

7. Point the refractometer toward a light source and observe the level where the dark and the light portion meet. Record the urine's specific gravity on the work sheet and in the patient's chart.
Ensures accuracy of reporting

8. Rinse the refractometer clean with distilled water, and dry it with gauze or a cleansing wipe.
Prepares the instrument for the next use

9. Clean the work area and dispose of waste properly. Remove PPE gown, gloves, and face shield, and wash your hands.
Ensures a clean work environment; prevents the spread of pathogens

Procedure Notes:

You Need to Know:

- Quality controls must be performed daily and recorded in the appropriate quality control record. Use distilled water for the negative control and a manufactured control or NaCl for the positive control. Follow office procedures for ensuring accurate calibration.
- The prism is delicate; avoid scratching it as you clean it.
- The entire refractometer must be free of residue before beginning the procedure.
- Refractometers vary. Read the manufacturer's instructions before beginning the test.
- If the specific gravity for the test is greater than the highest marking on the refractometer (usually 1.035), dilute the specimen with distilled water (10 drops of water to 10 drops of urine) in a glass tube. Mix, read the results, and multiply by 2.

21

Document on the Patient's Chart:
- Date and time
- Performance of procedure
- Testing results
- Action taken (if any)
- Signature

EXAMPLE

7/5/04	Urine specimen collected and
0745	tested for specific gravity using
	refractometer. Results: 1.005.
	—William Bendt, CMA

- If urine has been refrigerated, allow it to reach room temperature because cold affects specific gravity readings.

The specific gravity of urine can also be determined using a urinometer.

Procedure 21-5

Determining Specific Gravity (SG) of Urine Using a Urinometer

1. Assemble this equipment:
   - Patient's labeled urine specimen
   - Urinometer with cylinder
   - Patient report form
   - Cleansing wipe or clean paper towel

2. Follow these Standard Precautions.

21

3. Wash your hands and put on PPE gown.

4. Verify that the names on the specimen container and the laboratory form are the same.

5. Make sure the urinometer is clean before beginning. Use distilled water and a wipe or paper towel to wipe the inside of the cylinder and urinometer so that they are free of lint and moisture.

6. Add the patient's well-mixed, room-temperature urine specimen to the two-thirds mark in the cylinder. Add the urinometer to the cylinder with a spinning motion. *Frees the urinometer to reflect an accurate reading*

7. Read the specific gravity of the urine specimen from the urinometer scale. Observe the value from the bottom of the meniscus.

8. Record the value on the patient's report form and in the patient's chart.

9. Rinse with distilled water and wipe the urinometer dry after the testing procedure.

10. Clean the work area and dispose of waste properly. Remove gown, gloves, and face shield. Wash your hands. *Ensures a clean work environment; prevents spread of pathogens*

Procedure Notes:

You Need to Know:

- Quality controls must be performed daily and recorded in the appropriate quality control record. Use distilled water for the negative control and NaCl for the positive control. Follow office policies and procedures for ensuring accurate calibration.
- A sufficient amount of the specimen is needed for the urinometer to float accurately. If not enough urine is provided, report quantity not sufficient (QNS) and notify the physician.
- To avoid a QNS sample, check the quantity of urine before the patient leaves the area.
- Urinometers vary. Read the manufacturer's instructions before beginning the test.
- Urine must be at room temperature for accurate test results. Very warm urine tests falsely low; cold urine tests falsely high.
- Urinometers also are known as hydrometers.

21

Document on the Patient's Chart:

- Date and time
- Performance of procedure
- Testing results
- Action taken (if any)
- Signature

	Note: See charting example for Pro-
	cedure 21-1: Obtaining a Clean Catch
	Midstream (CCMS) Urine Specimen.

Urine can be tested using a chemical strip.

Procedure 21-6

Performing Chemical Reagent Strip Analysis

1. Assemble this equipment:
   - Patient's labeled urine specimen
   - Chemical strip (such as Multistix or Chemstrip)
   - Manufacturer's color-comparison chart
   - Stopwatch or timer

2. Follow these Standard Precautions.

3. Wash your hands and put on gloves and PPE gown.
   Reduces exposure to pathogens

4. Verify that the names on the specimen container and the laboratory form are the same.
   Avoids errors in identification

5. Mix patient's urine by gently swirling the covered container.
   Resuspends particulate matter into urine

6. Remove the reagent strip from its container and replace the lid to prevent deterioration of strips by humidity.

21

7. Immerse the reagent strip in the urine completely, then immediately remove it, sliding the side edge of the strip along the lip of the urine container to remove excess urine from the pads.

Prevents leaching colors from prolonged exposure to urine

8. Compare the reagent pad areas to the color chart, determining results at the intervals stated by the manufacturer. For example, glucose is read at 30 seconds. To determine results, examine that pad 30 seconds after dipping and compare with the color chart for glucose.

9. Read all reactions, and record the results for each reaction on the work sheet.

Adheres to strict, time-sensitive testing protocol

10. Discard the reagent strips in the proper receptacle. Discard urine unless more testing is required.

11. Clean the work area. Remove PPE gown. Wash your hands.

Ensures a clean work environment; prevents spread of pathogens

Procedure Notes:

WARNING!

Do not remove the desiccant packet in the strip container because it ensures that the strips are minimally affected by moisture. Be aware that the desiccant is toxic and should be discarded appropriately after all the strips have been used.

You Need to Know:

- The manufacturer's color-comparison chart is assigned a lot number that must match the lot number of the strips used for testing. Record this in the quality assurance/quality control (QA/QC) log.
- False-positive and false-negative results are possible. Review the manufacturer's package insert accompanying the strips to learn about factors that may give false results and how to avoid them.

21

Document on the Patient's Chart:

- Date and time
- Performance of procedure
- Testing results
- Action taken (if any)
- Your signature

EXAMPLE

	Note: See charting example for Pro-
	cedure 21-1: Obtaining a Clean Catch
	Midstream (CCMS) Urine Specimen.

- Aspirin may cause a false-positive result for ketones. Document whether the patient is taking aspirin or other medications. If the patient is taking Pyridium, do not use a chemical strip for testing.
- Outdated materials may give inaccurate results.

How can you test for glycosuria?

Procedure 21-7

Performing a Copper Reduction Test (Clinitest) for Glucose

1. Assemble this equipment:
   - Patient's labeled urine specimen
   - Positive and negative controls
   - Clinitest tablets (tightly sealed or new bottle)
   - 16 × 125-mm glass test tubes
   - Test tube rack
   - Transfer pipettes
   - Distilled water
   - Stopwatch or timer
   - Clinitest five-drop color-comparison chart
   - Daily sample log
   - Patient report form or data form

   Glass test tubes are used because plastic test tubes would melt from the heat generated by the reaction.

21

Performing a Copper Reduction Test for Glucose

2. Follow these Standard Precautions.

3. Wash hands and put on PPE gown, gloves, and face shield.
Reduces exposure to pathogens

4. Identify the patient's specimen to be tested, and record patient and sample information on the daily log.
Complies with QA/QC requirements

5. Record the patient's name or identification information, catalog and lot numbers for all test and control materials, and expiration dates on report or data form.
Complies with QA/QC requirements

6. Label test tubes with patient sample identification or as controls and place in the test tube rack.
Prevents misidentification

7. Using a transfer pipette, add 10 drops of distilled water to each labeled test tube in the rack. Add drops by holding the dropper vertically to ensure proper delivery.

8. Add five drops of the patient's urine or control sample to appropriately labeled tubes, using a different transfer pipette for each.
Prevents diluting urine with water or contaminating water with urine

9. Open Clinitest bottle and shake a Clinitest tablet into the lid without touching it. Then drop the tablet from the lid into the sample in the test tube rack. Repeat for all patient and control samples being tested.
Prevents a false test result

10. Observe reactions in the test tubes as the mixture boils. After the reaction stops, wait 15 seconds, then gently shake the test tubes.
Mixes the contents for reading results

21

11. Compare results for the patient specimen and controls with the five-drop method color chart immediately after shaking.
Ensures testing accuracy

Performing a Copper Reduction Test for Glucose

12. Clean and disinfect the work area and dispose of all
    waste properly. Remove gown, gloves, and face shield.
    Wash your hands.
    Ensures a clean work environment; prevents spread of pathogens

Procedure Notes:

WARNING!

*Always use glass test tubes, never plastic. Do not touch the test tube
bottoms because they become very hot during the test reaction.*

You Need to Know:

- Watch during boiling reaction to see if the tube contents pass
  through all of the colors on the five-drop color chart and result in
  a final color that reflects a lower score than one seen during the
  reaction. This is known as "pass-through phenomenon" and should
  be reported as "exceeds 2%." If your office requires a precise
  quantitative result on samples that show the pass-through phenomenon, perform the two-drop method. (Refer to the Clinitest package insert and use the two-drop color chart for interpretation.)
- Clinitest may be used as a test in the following situations:
  —When dipstick urine tests for glucose cannot be interpreted
  —For children under age 2 who are having urine tested for prob-
    lems with glucose metabolism (regardless of dipstick result)
- If positive or negative controls do not give expected results, the
  test is invalid and must be repeated.
- Certain medications (ascorbic acid) and reducing substances other
  than glucose (galactose and lactose) may give false-positive results.
  If this occurs, further testing is necessary.
- Keep the Clinitest bottle tightly capped at all times because mois-
  ture causes the tablets to deteriorate, thus affecting test results.

21

Performing a Nitroprusside Reaction for Ketones

Document on the Patient's Chart:

- Date and time
- Performance of procedure
- Testing results
- Action taken (if any)
- Your signature

	EXAMPLE
2/9/04	Patient diagnosed IDDM on last
1745	visit. Urine specimen collected.
	Urine tested for glucose with
	Clinitest. Results: 4+.
	—Keshaun Bowen, CMA

Does your patient have ketones in her urine?

Procedure 21-8

Performing a Nitroprusside Reaction (Acetest) for Ketones

1. Assemble this equipment:
   - Patient's labeled urine specimen
   - Acetest tablet
   - White filter paper
   - Plastic transfer pipette
   - Manufacturer's color-comparison chart
   - Stopwatch or timer

2. Follow these Standard Precautions.

3. Wash your hands and put on PPE gown.
   Reduces exposure to pathogens

21

4. Verify that the names on the specimen container and the laboratory form are the same.

5. Place an Acetest tablet on the filter paper by shaking one into the bottle cap and dispensing it onto the paper. Replace cap.
Prevents contamination of tablet or bottle contents

6. Using a transfer pipette, place one drop of well-mixed urine on top of the tablet.
Begins the reaction

7. Wait 30 seconds for the complete reaction. Compare tablet color with the color chart, and record the results on the work sheet and patient log form. The degree of purple color indicates the ketone concentration in the urine.
Provides accuracy in testing

8. Properly care for and dispose of equipment and supplies. Clean the work area. Remove gown, gloves, and face shield. Wash your hands.
Ensures a clean work environment; prevents spread of pathogens

Procedure Notes:

You Need to Know:

* If the urine is red in color, you may have trouble reading the reaction properly. Pour off a representative sample of urine (aliquot) into a test tube and centrifuge as you would for preparing a urine sediment (Procedure 21-11). If the red color is caused by intact red blood cells (RBC), the centrifuged urine should have a normal color. Use a drop of supernatant to test.

21

Performing an Acid Precipitation Test for Protein

Document on the Patient's Chart:
- Date and time
- Performance of procedure
- Testing results
- Action taken (if any)
- Your signature

9/2/04	Urine specimen collected and
1645	tested for ketones. Results
	showed large amount. Dr. Wendt
	notified.
	—Erik Smith, CMA

Does the physician suspect increased protein in a patient's urine?

Procedure 21-9

Performing an Acid Precipitation Test for Protein

1. Assemble this equipment:
   - Patient's labeled urine specimen
   - Positive and negative controls
   - 3% sulfosalicylic acid (SSA) solution
   - Clear glass test tubes
   - Test tube rack
   - Transfer pipettes
   - Centrifuge equipment
   - Stopwatch or timer
   - Daily sample log
   - Patient report form or data form

2. Follow these Standard Precautions.

3. Wash your hands and put on impervious gown, gloves, and face shield.
   Reduces exposure to pathogens

4. Identify patient's specimen to be tested, and record patient and sample information on the daily log.
   Avoids errors; complies with QA/QC requirements

5. Record patient's name or identification information, catalog and lot numbers for all test and control materials, and expiration dates on report or data form.
   Complies with QA/QC requirements

6. Label test tubes with patient sample identification or as controls and place them in test tube rack.
   Avoids misidentification

7. Centrifuge urine at 1,500 rpm for 5 minutes (Procedure 21-11).

8. Add 1 to 3 mL of supernatant urine (top portion of spun urine) or control sample to appropriately labeled tube in rack. Repeat for all samples and controls, using a clean transfer pipette for each.
   Avoids contamination of test results

9. Add an equal amount of 3% SSA solution to sample quantity in each tube. Use a clean transfer pipette for each addition if your 3% SSA solution does not have a repeating dispenser.
   Reduces errors in testing

10. Mix the contents of the tubes and let stand for a minimum of 2 minutes but no longer than 10 minutes. Use a stopwatch or timer to make sure you perform the next step within the appropriate time frame.
    Provides for accuracy in testing

11. Mix contents of tubes again, then observe the degree of turbidity seen in each test tube and score as follows:
    - Negative: No turbidity or cloudiness; urine remains clear
    - Trace: Slight turbidity
    - 1+: Turbidity with no precipitation (print on a page held behind tube is visible)
    - 2+: Heavy turbidity with fine granulation

21

Performing an Acid Precipitation Test for Protein

Document on the Patient's Chart:
- Date and time
- Performance of procedure
- Testing results
- Action taken (if any)
- Your signature

EXAMPLE

7/7/04	Urine specimen collected and
0830	tested for protein using acid pre-
	cipitation test. Results: 3+.
	—Gail Trembly, CMA

- 3+: Heavy turbidity with granulation and flakes
- 4+: Clumps of precipitated protein

12. Clean work area and dispose of all waste properly. Remove gown, gloves, and face shield. Wash your hands.
Ensures a clean work environment; prevents spread of pathogens

Procedure Notes:

You Need to Know:
- This is a confirmatory test used for specimens with dipstick urine test results greater than trace value for protein.
- If supernatant from centrifuged urine is not used or the specimen is not mixed well with reagent after centrifugation, a false-positive result may occur.
- If positive and negative controls do not give expected results, the test is invalid and must be repeated.
- The specimen may be matched against a McFarland standard to decrease the degree of subjective interpretation.

21

What urine test may be used to help determine a patient's liver function?

Procedure 21-10

Performing a Diazo Tablet Test (Ictotest) for Bilirubin

1. Assemble this equipment:
   - Patient's labeled urine specimen
   - Ictotest (diazo) tablets
   - Ictotest white mats
   - Clean paper towel
   - Transfer pipette
   - Stopwatch or timer

2. Follow these Standard Precautions.

3. Wash your hands and put on PPE gown, gloves, and face shield.
   Reduces exposure to pathogens

4. Verify that the names on the specimen container and the laboratory form are the same.

5. Place an Ictotest white mat on a clean, dry paper towel.
   Provides a testing surface

6. Using a clean transfer pipette, add 10 drops of the patient's urine to the center of the mat.

7. Shake a tablet into the bottle cap and dispense onto the center of the mat. Do not touch the tablet with your hands because doing so may cause a false-positive result.
   Avoids contaminating tablet

8. Recap the bottle immediately.
   Prevents deterioration of bottle contents

9. Using a clean transfer pipette, place one drop of water on the tablet and wait 5 seconds.

10. Add another drop of water to the tablet so that the solution formed by the first drop runs onto the mat.
    Allows diazo chemical to react with urine

21

Performing a Diazo Tablet Test for Bilirubin

Document on the Patient's Chart:
- Date and time
- Performance of procedure
- Testing results
- Action taken (if any)
- Your signature

5/4/04	Urine specimen collected and
1635	tested for bilirubin using diazo
	test. Results: positive.
	—Kim Opal, CMA

11. Within 60 seconds observe for either a blue or purple color on the mat around the tablet. Either color indicates a positive result.

12. Clean the work area and dispose of waste properly. Remove gown, gloves, and face shield. Wash your hands.
Ensures a clean work environment; prevents spread of pathogens

Procedure Notes:

You Need to Know:
- Quality controls must be performed daily and recorded appropriately. Follow office policies and procedures for ensuring compliance with QA/QC requirements.
- Protect the tablets from exposure to light, heat, and moisture to prevent deterioration.
- The specimen should be free of Pyridium, chlorpromazine, or other drugs that interfere with color interpretation.
- If the urine is red in color, it may be difficult to read the reaction properly. Pour a representative sample (aliquot) of the urine into a urine tube or test tube and centrifuge as you would for preparing

21

urine sediment (Procedure 21-11). Use 10 drops of supernatant in step 6.

- Moisture on the paper towel may cause a false result.
- A pink or red color indicates a negative result.

Do you need to test the concentrated particulate matter in the urine specimen?

Procedure 21-11

Preparing a Urine Sediment

1. Assemble this equipment:
    - Patient's labeled urine specimen
    - Urine centrifuge tubes
    - Transfer pipette
    - Centrifuge (1,500 to 2,000 rpm)

2. Follow these Standard Precautions.

3. Wash your hands and put on PPE gown, gloves, and face shield.
    Reduces exposure to pathogens

4. Verify that the names on the specimen container and the laboratory form are the same.

5. Pour 10 to 15 mL of the patient's well-mixed urine into a labeled centrifuge tube (or a standardized system tube). Cap the tube with a plastic cap or film.

6. Place the labeled urine tube in the centrifuge and balance it with another tube (filled to the same level with water or another patient's urine).
    Prevents damage to centrifuge due to imbalance of rotor

7. Close centrifuge cover and set it to spin at 1,500 rpm for 5 minutes.
    Ensures that cellular and particulate matter is pushed to the bottom of the tube

8. When the centrifuge has stopped, remove the tubes. Save the supernatant if it is to be tested. Remove the caps and pour off the supernatant, leaving a small por-

21

tion of supernatant (0. 5 to 1. 0 mL). Resuspend the
sediment by flicking the tube with your finger, aspirating sample up and down with a transfer pipette, or
following manufacturer's directions for standardized
system.

Prepares concentrated urine for microscopic examination

9. Properly care for and dispose of equipment and supplies. Clean the work area. Remove gown, gloves, and
shield. Wash your hands.

Ensures a clean work environment; prevents spread of pathogens

Procedure Notes:

You Need to Know:

- If the urine is to be tested by chemical reagent strip, perform the
  dip test before spinning the urine.
- Preparing a urine for sediment with less than 3 mL is not recommended because that is not enough urine to create a true sediment. However, some patients are unable to provide a large
  amount of urine. In such cases, document the volume on the chart
  under sediment to ensure proper interpretation of results.
- Check the centrifuge periodically to ensure that the speed and
  timing are correct. Document this information on the maintenance
  log.

**If the components of a urinary sample must
be identified, use this procedure.**

Procedure 21-12

21

Preparing Urine for Microscopic Examination

1. Assemble this equipment:
- Patient's labeled urine tube
- Transfer pipette
- Microscope
- Lens cleaner
- Lens paper

- Glass slide
- Coverslip
- Standardized sediment slide (if applicable)

2. Follow these Standard Precautions.

3. Wash your hands and put on PPE gown, gloves, and face shield.
Reduces exposure to pathogens

4. Verify that the names on the specimen container and the laboratory form are the same.

5. Using a centrifuged urine specimen (Procedure 21-11), make sure the sediment is well-mixed with the remaining 1 mL of urine.
Ensures proper mixing for accurate results

6. Using the transfer pipette, place one drop of the urine mixture onto a clean glass slide or into the chamber of the standardized slide.
Distributes sediment for examination

7. Place a coverslip over the drop of urine if using the glass slide.
Secures specimen to slide for viewing

8. Place the slide on the microscope stage between the holding clips. Using the 10× objective, focus until the sediment structures (cells and so forth) become clear.
Ensures that no components are overlooked

9. Examine the edges of the specimen for casts, scanning about 10 to 15 fields. If a cast is present, use the 40× objective to identify the type (waxy, granular, hyaline, white blood cell [WBC], RBC). To report the number of casts present, take the average seen under the low-power, 10× objective. Example: 0 to 1 hyaline cast per low-power field (LPF). Record any casts observed on the work sheet and laboratory form.
Ensures accuracy in reporting

21

10. Scan the slide using the 40× objective for about 10 to 15 fields. Record the average number of RBC, WBC, and epithelial cells observed on the work sheet and laboratory form.

11. Observe the presence of bacteria, mucus, crystals, sperm, yeast, and *Trichomonas vaginalis* using the 40× objective for 10 fields. Use references located in the laboratory area to identify structures as needed. Record the average number or amount observed on the work sheet and laboratory form.

12. Report your observations as follows:
    - Epithelial: Rare, few, moderate, many
    - Casts: Number and type per LPF
    - Mucus: Trace, 1+, 2+, 3+, 4+
    - WBC: Lowest number and highest number seen in 10 fields per high-power field (HPF). Example: 0 to 5 WBC/HPF.
    - RBC: Lowest number and highest number seen in 10 fields per HPF. Example: 2 to 10 RBC/HPF.
    - Bacteria: Trace, 1+, 2+, 3+, 4+
    - Crystals, yeast, sperm, *Trichomonas:* Few, moderate, many, and type
      Note: 1+ = few in some fields; 2+ = few in all fields; 3+ = many in all fields; 4+ = too numerous to count (TNTC).

13. Clean the work area and dispose of waste properly. Remove gown, gloves, and face shield. Wash your hands.
    Ensures a clean work environment; prevents spread of pathogens

Procedure Notes:

21

Document on the Patient's Chart:

- Date and time
- Performance of procedure
- Testing results
- Action taken (if any)
- Your signature

EXAMPLE

9/5/04	Microscopic examination of urine.
1235	Results: 8 WBC/HPF and 1 RBC
	cast/LPF.
	—Hugh Krent, CMA

You Need to Know:

- According to CLIA regulations, medical assistants may perform the microscopic examination up to step 8 to have the slide in focus for the physician and to point out types of sediment. If the medical assistant has been trained to complete the procedure, steps 9 through 11 may be completed.
- The 10X objective is used to focus and scan; the 40X or 45X objective is used to identify components.

21

Rapid Test Procedures

Note: There are many different types of rapid test kits available on the market today. Be sure to follow specific manufacturer's instructions for each kit.

The following procedures are for a few of the rapid test kits on the market today.

Does your patient have infectious mononucleosis?

Procedure 22-1

Performing a Mononucleosis Test

1. Assemble this equipment:
   - Patient's labeled specimen (whole blood, plasma, or serum, depending on the kit)
   - Mononucleosis kit (slide or card, controls, reagents, capillary tubes, bulb, and stirrers)
   - Stopwatch or timer
   - Saline, test tubes, pipettes (if titration is required)

2. Follow these Standard Precautions.

3. Verify that the name on the specimen container and the laboratory form are the same.

4. Put on gloves, PPE gown, and face shield.
   Reduces exposure to pathogens

5. Label the slide or card (depending on the type of kit used) with the patient's name, positive control, and negative control. One circle or space is provided per patient and control.
Ensures accurate documentation

6. Place the rubber bulb on the capillary tube and aspirate the patient's specimen up to the marked line. Dispense the sample in the middle of the circle labeled with the patient's name. Avoid air bubbles to ensure accurate results.
Ensures that specimen is delivered properly

7. Gently mix the positive control. Using the capillary tube, aspirate the positive control up to the marked line. Dispense the control in the middle of the circle labeled positive control. Avoid air bubbles.
Adheres to quality assurance/quality control (QA/QC) requirements

8. Mix the latex reagent and add one drop to each circle or space (patient sample, positive control, negative control). Avoid splashing the reagents, which can result in cross-contamination and incorrect results.
Ensures testing accuracy

9. Using a clean stirrer for each test, mix the reagent with the patient sample and controls. Mix only one circle at a time, keeping within each circle. Going outside of the circle may lead to cross contamination and incorrect results.
Ensures testing accuracy

10. Gently rock the slide for 2 minutes and observe for agglutination (clumping). Testing time may vary if using a disposable card.

11. Verify the results of the controls before documenting the patient's results. Log controls and patient information on the work sheet.

12. Read the kit's instructions if titration is required.

13. Clean the work area and dispose of waste properly. Wash the slide thoroughly with bleach and rinse with water before using again. Remove gown, gloves, and shield. Wash your hands.
Ensures a clean work environment; prevents spread of pathogens

22

Document on the Patient's Chart:

- Date and time
- Performance of procedure
- Testing results
- Action taken (if any)
- Your signature

EXAMPLE

8/1/04	Mono spot = neg on serum.
0930	Dr. Royal notified.
	—Nyla Pressman, CMA

Procedure Notes:

You Need to Know:

- Kits vary depending on the manufacturer. Read instructions carefully before beginning the procedure.
- Depending on the kit used, the specimen required may be whole blood, plasma, or serum.
- Ensure that the materials in the kit are at room temperature before beginning the procedure.
- Controls for test kits are usually run once per day or kit. Follow office policies and procedures for ensuring testing accuracy and maintaining quality control.
- Controls are needed when performing a titration.

How can you determine if your patient is pregnant?

22

Procedure 22-2

Performing a hCG Pregnancy Test

I. Assemble this equipment:
  - Patient's labeled specimen (plasma, serum, or urine, depending on the kit)

- Human chorionic gonadotropin (hCG) pregnancy kit (test pack and transfer pipettes; kit contents vary by manufacturer)
- hCG-positive and hCG -negative control (different controls may be needed when testing urine)
- Timer

2. Follow these Standard Precautions.

3. Verify that the names on the specimen container and the laboratory form are the same.

4. Put on gloves, impervious gown, and face shield.
Reduces exposure to pathogens

5. Label the test pack (depending on type of kit) with the patient's name, positive control, and negative control. Use one test pack per patient and control.
Avoids misidentification

6. Note in the patient's information and in the control log whether you are using urine, plasma, or serum for testing. Kit and controls must be at room temperature for testing.
Ensures testing accuracy

7. Aspirate the patient's specimen using the transfer pipette and place three drops (180 mL) on the sample well of the test pack labeled with the patient's name.
Adheres to testing protocol

8. Aspirate the positive control using a new transfer pipette and place three drops (180 mL) on the sample well of the test pack labeled positive control. Avoid splashing to eliminate cross-contamination.
Observes QA/QC standards

9. Aspirate the negative control using the transfer pipette and place three drops (180 mL) on the sample well of the test pack labeled negative control. Avoid splashing to eliminate cross-contamination.
Observes QA/QC standards

22

Document on the Patient's Chart:

- Date and time
- Performance of procedure
- Testing results
- Action taken (if any)
- Your signature

EXAMPLE

1/14/04	Pt. presented complaining of late
1615	period. LMP: 11/22/03. Complained
	of nausea in the AM, breast ten-
	derness. Urine sample positive for
	pregnancy. Dr. Wong in to examine
	pt. Pregnancy brochures explained
	to pt. RTC 2/14/04.
	—Alison Jung, CMA

10. Report the results when the "End of Assay" window is red. This takes approximately 7 minutes for serum samples and 4 minutes for urine samples. Check to verify controls before reporting the results.
Ensures that testing is complete

11. Record controls and patient information on the work sheet and log form.

12. Clean the work area and dispose of waste properly. Remove gown, gloves, and shield. Wash your hands.
Ensures a clean work environment; prevents spread of pathogens

22

Procedure Notes:

You Need to Know:

- Kits vary depending on the manufacturer. Read instructions carefully before beginning the procedure.
- Depending on the kit used, the specimen required may be plasma, serum, or urine.
- Controls for test kits are usually run once per day or kit. Follow office policies and procedures for ensuring testing accuracy and maintaining quality control.
- Repeat the test if the "End of Assay" window does not appear and if the controls do not work.

Stop the spread of strep by quickly identifying a positive throat culture.

Procedure 22-3

Performing a Group A Rapid Strep Test

1. Assemble this equipment:
   - Patient's labeled throat culture (use a Culturette with two swabs provided)
   - Group A strep kit (controls may be included, depending on the kit)
   - Timer
   - Beta strep agar
   - Bacitracin disks

2. Follow these Standard Precautions.

3. Verify that the name on the specimen container and the laboratory form are the same.

4. Put on gloves, PPE gown, and face shield.
   Reduces exposure to pathogens

5. Label one extraction tube with the patient's name, another with the positive control, and one with the negative control.
   Ensures testing accuracy

6. Follow the directions for the kit. Add the appropriate reagents and drops to each of the extraction tubes.

22

Avoid splashing and use the correct number of drops.
Adheres to testing guidelines

7. Insert the patient's swab (one of the two swabs present) into the labeled extraction tube. If only one culture swab was submitted, first swab a beta strep agar plate, then use the swab for the rapid strep test.
Begins testing process without contaminating culture specimen

8. Add the appropriate controls to each of the labeled extraction tubes.
Begins chemical reaction for proper control results

9. Set timer for appropriate time.
Ensures testing accuracy

10. Add the appropriate reagent and drops to each of the extraction tubes.
Continues testing protocol

11. Use the swab to mix the reagents, then press out any excess fluid remaining on the swab by placing your fingers on the outside of the extraction tube while pinching the swab against the inside of the tube.
Deposits maximum amount of substance to be tested

12. Add three drops from the well-mixed extraction tube to the sample window of the strep A test unit labeled with the patient's name. Do the same for each control with drops from the appropriate extraction tubes.
Ensures accurate results

13. Set the timer for the appropriate time.
Ensures that timing protocols are followed

14. Be aware that a positive result appears as a line in the result window within 5 minutes. An internal control is present in the strep A test unit; if a line appears in the control window, the test is valid.

15. Verify results of the controls before recording test results. Log the controls and the patient information on the work sheet.
Ensures accuracy of reporting

16. Clean the work area and dispose of waste properly. Remove gown, gloves, and shield. Wash your hands.
Ensures a clean work environment; prevents spread of pathogens

22

Document on the Patient's Chart:
- Date and time
- Performance of procedure
- Testing results
- Action taken (if any)
- Your signature

EXAMPLE

6/8/04	Pt. complained of sore throat
1115	× 2 days. Group A rapid strep
	test positive. Dr. Harrison notified.
	—Lyn Zachary, RMA

Procedure Notes:

You Need to Know:
- Kits vary depending on the manufacturer. Read instructions carefully before beginning the procedure.
- Controls for test kits are usually run once per day or kit. Follow office policies and procedures for ensuring testing accuracy and maintaining quality control.
- Depending on laboratory protocol, you may need to culture all negative rapid strep screens on beta strep agar. A bacitracin disk may be added to the first quadrant while setting up or after 24 hours if a beta hemolytic colony appears. A culture is more sensitive than a rapid immunoassay test.
- Beta strep agar and bacitracin need to come to room temperature before being used.
- Read a negative result at exactly 5 minutes to avoid a false-negative result.

22

Metric Measurement Equivalents

Unit	Abbreviation	Metric Equivalent	U.S. Equivalent
Units of Weight			
Kilogram	kg	1000 g	2.2 lb
Gram*	g	1000 mg	0.035 oz; 28.5 g/oz
Milligram	mg	$\frac{1}{1000}$ mm; 0.001 g	
Microgram	μg	$\frac{1}{1000}$ mg; 0.001 mg	
Units of Length			
Kilometer	km	1000 meters	0.62 miles; 1.6 km/mile
Meter*	m	100 cm; 1000 mm	39.4 inches; 1.1 yards
Centimeter	cm	$\frac{1}{100}$ m; 0.01 m	0.39 inches; 2.5 cm/inch
Millimeter	mm	$\frac{1}{1000}$ m; 0.001 m	0.039 inches; 25 mm/inch
Micrometer	μm	$\frac{1}{1000}$ mm; 0.001 mm	
Units of Volume			
Liter*	L	1000 mL	1.06 qt
Deciliter	dL	$\frac{1}{10}$ L; 0.1 L	
Milliliter	mL	$\frac{1}{1000}$ L; 0.001 L	0.034 oz., 29.4 mL/oz
Microliter	μL	$\frac{1}{1000}$ mL; 0.001 mL	

Reprinted with permission from Memmler RL, Cohen BJ, Wood DL. The Human Body in Health and Disease, 8th ed. Philadelphia: Lippincott-Raven, 1996.
*Basic unit.

Appendix II

Appendix II

Abbreviations Commonly Used in Documentation

Abbreviation	Meaning	Abbreviation	Meaning
ā	before	gm	gram
abd	abdomen	gr	grain
ac	before meals	gt/gtt	drop/drops
ADL	activities of daily living	"H," SC, or sub q	hypodermic or subcutaneous
ad lib	as needed	h	hour
adm	admitted, admission	HOB	head of bed
		h.s.	bedtime (hour of sleep)
amp	ampule		
ant.	anterior	Hx	history
AP	anterior-posterior	I & O	intake & output
ax.	axillary	IM	intramuscular
b.i.d.	twice a day	IV	intravenous
BP	blood pressure	kg	kilogram
BR	bed rest	KVO	keep vein open
BRP	bathroom privileges	L	left, liter
		lat	lateral
C	Celsius	MAE	moves all extremities
c̄	with		
caps	capsule	mg	milligram
CC	chief complaint	ml, mL	milliliter (1 mL = 1 cc)
cc	cubic centimeter (1 cc = 1 mL)		
		NAD	no apparent distress
c/o	complains of		
CVP	central venous pressure	NG	nasogastric
		NKDA	no known drug allergies
CPX	complete physical examination		
		noct.	nocturnal
Cx	canceled	NPO	nothing by mouth
D/C	discontinue	os	mouth
disch; DC	discharge	OOB	out of bed
drsg	dressing	oz	ounce
dr	dram	p̄	after
elix	elixir	p.c.	after meals
ext	extract or external	post	posterior
		prep	preparation
F	Fahrenheit	pm	when necessary
Fx	fracture, fractional	p.r.n.	as needed

Appendix II

Abbreviations Commonly Used in Documentation—cont'd

Abbreviation	Meaning	Abbreviation	Meaning
pt.	patient	VS	vital signs
q̄, q	every	VSS	vital signs stable
q̄ 2 (3, 4, etc.) hours	every 2 (3, 4, etc.) hours	W/C	wheelchair
qd	every day	WNL	within normal limits
qh	every hour		
q.i.d.	four times a day	**Selected Abbreviations Used**	
q.o.d.	every other day	**for Specific Descriptions**	
q.s.	quantity sufficient	AKA	above-knee amputation
R	right	ASCVD	arteriosclerotic cardiovascular disease
R/O	rule out		
ROM	range of motion		
r/s	rescheduled	BKA	below-knee amputation
s̄	without		
SBA	stand by assistance	ca	cancer
SC	subcutaneous	chest clear to A & P	chest clear to auscultation & percussion
SL	sublingual		
SOB	shortness of breath		
sol, soln	solution		
spec	specimen	CMS	circulation movement sensation
s/p	status post		
sp. gr.	specific gravity	CNS	central nervous system
S.S.E.	soapsuds enema		
ss	one-half	DJD	degenerative joint disease
STAT	immediately		
tab	tablet	DOE	dyspnea on exertion
t.i.d.	three times a day		
tinct or tr.	tincture	DTs	delirium tremens
TKO	to keep open	D₅W	5% dextrose in water
TPN	total parenteral nutrition hyperalimentation		
		FUO	fever of unknown origin
TPR	temperature, pulse, respiration	GB	gallbladder
		GI	gastrointestinal
tsp	teaspoon	GYN	gynecology
TO	telephone order	H₂O₂	hydrogen peroxide
TWE	tap water enema	HA	hyperalimentation headache
VO	verbal order		

Appendix II

Abbreviations Commonly Used in Documentation—cont'd

Abbreviation	Meaning	Abbreviation	Meaning
HCVD	hypertensive cardiovascular disease	OT	occupational therapy
HEENT	head, ear, eye, nose, throat	PE	physical examination
HVD	hypertensive vascular disease	PERRLA	pupils equal, round, & react to light and accommodation
ICU	intensive care unit		
I & D	incision and drainage	PID	pelvic inflammatory disease
LLE	left lower extremity	PI	present illness
LLQ	left lower quadrant	PM & R	physical medicine & rehabilitation
LOC	level of consciousness; laxatives of choice	Psych	psychology; psychiatric
LMP	last menstrual period	PT	physical therapy
		RL (or LR)	Ringer's lactate; lactated Ringer's
LUE	left upper extremity	RLE	right lower extremity
LUQ	left upper quadrant	RLQ	right lower quadrant
MI	myocardial infarction	RR, PAR, PACU	recovery room, post-anesthesia room, post-anesthesia care unit
Neuro	neurology; neurosurgery		
NS	normal saline		
Nys.	nursery		
NWB	non–weight-bearing	RUE	right upper extremity
O.D.	right eye	RUQ	right upper quadrant
O.S.	left eye		
O.U.	each eye	Rx	prescription
OPD	outpatient department	STD	sexually transmitted disease
ORIF	open reduction internal fixation	STSG	split-thickness skin graft
Ortho	Orthopedics	Surg	surgery, surgical

Abbreviations Commonly Used in Documentation—cont'd

Abbreviation	Meaning	Abbreviation	Meaning
T & A	tonsillectomy & adenoidectomy	RBC	red blood cell
THR, TJR	total hip replacement; total joint replacement	UGI	upper gastro-intestinal x-ray
		UA	urinalysis
URI	upper respiratory infection	WBC	white blood cell

Commonly Used Symbols

Symbol	Meaning
>	greater than
<	less than
=	equal to
$\simeq$	approximately equal to
$\leq$	equal to or less than
$\geq$	equal to or greater than
$\uparrow$	increased
$\downarrow$	decreased
♀	female
♂	male
°	degree
#	number or pound
$\times$	times
@	at
+	positive
−	negative
$\pm$	positive or negative
F_1	first filial generation
F_2	second filial generation
PO_2	partial pressure of oxygen
PCO_2	partial pressure of carbon dioxide
:	ratio
∴	therefore
%	percent
2°	secondary to
△	change

Additional abbreviations:

Abbreviation	Meaning
UTI	urinary tract infection
vag	vaginal
WNWD	well-nourished, well-developed

Selected Abbreviations Related to Common Diagnostic Tests

Abbreviation	Meaning
BE	barium enema
BMR	basal metabolism rate
Ca^{++}	calcium
CAT	computed axial tomography
CBC	complete blood count
Cl^-	chloride
C & S	culture & sensitivity
Dx	diagnosis
ECG, EKG	electrocardiogram
EEG	electroencephalo-gram
FBS	fasting blood sugar
hct	hematocrit
Hgb	hemoglobin
IVP	intravenous pyelogram
K^+	potassium
LP	lumbar puncture
MRI	magnetic reso-nance imaging
Na^+	sodium

Reprinted with permission from Craven RF, Hirnle CJ. Human Health and Function, 2nd ed. Philadelphia: Lippincott-Raven, 1996.

Appendix III

Celsius–Fahrenheit Temperature Conversion Scale

Celsius to Fahrenheit	Fahrenheit to Celsius

Use the following formula to convert Celsius readings to Fahrenheit readings:

$$°F = 9/5°C + 32$$

For example, if the Celsius reading is 37°:

$°F = (9/5 \times 37) + 32$

$= 66.6 + 32$

$= 98.6°F$ (normal body temperature)

Use the following formula to convert Fahrenheit readings to Celsius readings:

$$°C = 5/9 \; (°F - 32)$$

For example, if the Fahrenheit reading is 68°:

$°C = 5/9 \; (68 - 32)$

$= 5/9 \times 36$

$= 20°C$ (a nice spring day)

Reprinted with permission from Memmler RL, Cohen BJ, Wood DL. The Human Body in Health and Disease, 8th ed. Philadelphia: Lippincott-Raven, 1996.

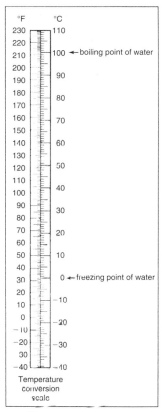

Appendix Figure III-I. Graphic comparison of Fahrenheit versus Celsius temperatures.

Bibliography

Andress A. Saunders Manual of Medical Office Management. Philadelphia: WB Saunders, 1966.

Androlina VF, et al. Mammographic Imaging: A Practical Guide. Philadelphia: JB Lippincott, 1992.

Bates B, et al. A Guide to Physical Examination and History Taking, 6th ed. Philadelphia: JB Lippincott, 1995.

Becklin KJ, Sunnarborg EM. Medical Office Procedures, 3rd ed. New York: Glencoe/McGraw-Hill, 1992.

Bishop ML, et al. Clinical Chemistry: Principles, Procedures, Correlations, 5th ed. Baltimore: Lippincott Williams & Wilkins, 2005.

Blood Borne Pathogens, OSHA Inst. 29CFR 1910.1030.

Boyer MJ. Math for Nurses: A Pocket Guide to Dosage Calculation and Drug Administration, 4th ed. Philadelphia: Lippincott-Raven, 1998.

Brown JL. Pediatric Telephone Medicine: Principles, Triage, and Advice, 2nd ed. Philadelphia: JB Lippincott, 1994.

Burton GG, et al. Respiratory Care: A Guide to Clinical Practice, 4th ed. Philadelphia: Lippincott-Raven, 1997.

Carpenito L. Handbook of Nursing Diagnosis, 7th ed. Philadelphia. Lippincott-Raven, 1997.

Craven RF, Hirnle CJ. Fundamentals of Nursing: Health and Human Function, 2nd ed. Philadelphia: Lippincott-Raven, 1996.

Cullinan AM. Producing Quality Radiographs, 2nd ed. Philadelphia: JB Lippincott, 1994.

DiDona NA., Marks MA. Introductory Maternal-Newborn Nursing. Philadelphia: Lippincott-Raven, 1996.

Fischbach F. A Manual of Laboratory and Diagnostic Tests, 5th ed. Philadelphia: Lippincott-Raven, 1996.

Fischbach F. Quick Reference for Laboratory and Diagnostic Tests, 2nd ed. Philadelphia: Lippincott-Raven, 1998.

Graff, Sister Laurine. A Handbook of Routine Urinalysis. Philadelphia: JB Lippincott, 1983.

Harwood-Nuss AL, Luten RC. Handbook of Emergency Medicine. Philadelphia: JB Lippincott, 1995.

Henke G. Med-Math: Dosage Calculation, Preparation and Administration, 2nd ed. Philadelphia: JB Lippincott, 1995.

Bibliography

Hodgkin JE, et al. Pulmonary Rehabilitation: Guidelines to Success, 2nd ed. Philadelphia: JB Lippincott, 1993.

Humphrey DD. Contemporary Medical Office Procedures. Cincinnati: South-Western Publishing, 1990.

Johnson JM, Johnson MW. Computerized Medical Office Management. Albany, NY: Delmar, 1994.

Jones SA, et al. Advanced Emergency Care for Paramedic Practice. Philadelphia: JB Lippincott, 1992.

Koneman EW, et al. Color Atlas and Textbook of Diagnostic Microbiology, 5th ed. Philadelphia: Lippincott-Raven, 1997.

Koneman EW, et al. Introduction to Diagnostic Microbiology. Philadelphia: JB Lippincott, 1994.

Lotspeich-Steininger C, et al. Clinical Hematology: Principles, Procedures and Correlations. Philadelphia: JB Lippincott, 1992.

McCall RE, Tankersley CM. Phlebotomy Essentials, 2nd ed. Philadelphia: Lippincott-Raven, 1998.

Nettina SM. The Lippincott Manual of Nursing Practice, 6th ed. Philadelphia: Lippincott-Raven, 1996.

Pillitteri A. Maternal and Child-Health Nursing: Care of the Child-Bearing and Child-Rearing Family, 2nd ed. Philadelphia: Lippincott-Raven, 1995.

Rappaport SI. Introduction to Hematology, 2nd ed. Philadelphia: JB Lippincott, 1987.

Reeder SJ, et al. Maternity Nursing: Family, Newborn and Women's Health Care, 18th ed. Philadelphia: Lippincott-Raven, 1997.

Rosdahl CB. Textbook of Basic Nursing, 6th ed. Philadelphia: Lippincott-Raven, 1995.

Scherer JC, Roach SS. Introductory Clinical Pharmacology, 5th ed. Philadelphia: JB Lippincott, 1995.

Scherer JC, Timby BK. Introductory Medical-Surgical Nursing, 6th ed. Philadelphia: JB Lippincott, 1995.

Scott JR, et al. Danforth's Obstetrics and Gynecology, 7th ed. Philadelphia: JB Lippincott, 1994.

Smeltzer SC, Bare BG. Brunner and Suddarth's Textbook of Medical-Surgical Nursing, 8th ed. Philadelphia: Lippincott-Raven, 1996.

Smith-Temple J, Johnson JY. Nurse's Guide to Clinical Procedures, 3rd ed. Philadelphia: Lippincott-Raven, 1998.

Strunk W, Jr, White EB. The Elements of Style, 3rd ed. New York: Macmillan, 1979.

Taylor C, et al. Fundamentals of Nursing: The Art and Science of Nursing Care, 3rd ed. Philadelphia: Lippincott-Raven, 1997.

Timby B. Fundamental Skills and Concepts in Patient Care, 6th ed. Philadelphia: Lippincott-Raven, 1996.

Torres LS. Basic Medical Techniques and Patient Care in Imaging Technology, 5th ed. Philadelphia: Lippincott-Raven, 1997.

Volk WA., et al. Essentials of Medical Microbiology, 5th ed. Philadelphia: Lippincott-Raven, 1996.

Walter JB. An Introduction to the Principles of Disease, 3rd ed. Philadelphia: JB Lippincott, 1992.

Index

Page numbers in *italics* denote figures; those followed by a "t" denote tables; those followed by a "b" denote boxed information.

Index

Index

Index

Index

Index